Infertility Saved My Life

Endorsements

I am in awe of the strength that Sarah shows through sharing her story. As someone who is also dealing with secondary infertility, has had multiple miscarriages, and gone through IVF, I can say without a doubt she captures the heartache and pain beautifully. It is so comforting and healing to connect with other women who share your same experiences. It is so important to get the message out to struggling women that we are not alone, and I thank her for doing so.

——**Lauren Flynn,** Singer/Songwriter for Folk/Pop Trio, OLIVIA FOX

Sarah masterfully interweaves her wisdom and phenomenal life story with tools and insights to rewire the brain from fear to love to facilitate healing and enhance mental and emotional well-being. Brilliant work!

——**Dr. Arayeh Norouzi,** Ph.D. in Psychology, Joyful Living Coach

Infertility Saved My Life: Healing PCOS from the Inside Out is truly a touching story containing life-changing insights. It is an absolute must-read for anyone struggling with PCOS, infertility or miscarriage. Sarah's voice is both vulnerable and powerful, and the exercises are a valuable bonus to this inspiring story.

——**Barbara Vercruysse,** Global Kindness Advocate, CEO and Founder of Barbara Vercruysse Coaching Institute, #1 Top 50 Global Thought Leaders on Mental Health

When we endure such complicated heartache we often feel isolated and alone. Sarah has given this a voice in a candid and supportive way. Not only does she share her inspiring story, but she opens her heart and mind to give the reader techniques and strategies to help and embrace the healing process.

——**Anita Thompson,** Heartache to Hope Podcast Host and HR/Marketing Professional

If I had been able to read *Infertility Saved My Life: Healing PCOS from the Inside Out* when I was going through my IVF treatments, things would have been easier. My journey would not have been filled with mixed emotions and such a deep pain. This is a masterpiece created with love and Sarah's wish to help women like us. Sarah's divine heart wrote this book, and her honesty and vulnerability moved me to tears. Her powerful story provides hope to those who are still waiting to become parents. I now feel empowered to find more joy and overcome future challenges.

—**Catherine B. Roy,** Business Coach

From the start, I could not put this down! Sarah continually encourages you to love yourself, motivates the reader to fight for themselves and makes you feel like you're living through these experiences right along with her. Her passion for the topic and relatability to the reader is remarkable. I really think this book can help boyfriends, husbands, fathers and even those in the medical field understand the struggle women with PCOS face. I encourage everyone to read *Infertility Saved My Life: Healing PCOS from the Inside Out.*

—**Robert Walls Jr,** CEO www.coasttocoastballers.com

A very personal and emotional story–extremely readable and full of practical information. This will help a LOT of people (both male and female) going through their own journeys.

—**Chris Lawson,** IVFDad Podcast

Sarah's story portrays the unbelievable challenges and emotional rollercoaster women go through living with PCOS, being diagnosed with secondary infertility, and going through miscarriages and failed IVF treatments. It is inspiring to see how, despite the fear and uncertainty, Sarah handles it with courage, resilience and keeps on holding on to hope. I believe the lessons and tools Sarah shares will help women walking a similar journey trust themselves, heal from within, and keep their focus on their well-being so they maximize their chances of conceiving.

—**Hala Dagher Chibani,** Soulful Business Strategist

I have stood in the exact same spaces as Sarah, both physically and emotionally. As I read, I reflected that along the journey to create new life, sometimes it is us who find a new life. Alongside infertility, Sarah covers the virtues of rest, recovery, healing and living life in all its fullness. A beautiful book. I loved it.

—**Aimée Knott,** Director Plucky People

Sarah's story is one of heartbreak and love. Told through vulnerability and understanding, she has turned her trauma into a shining light for those suffering from PCOS. *Infertility Saved My Life: Healing PCOS from the Inside Out* will help any family member struggling with infertility and PCOS in all areas of life including physically, mentally, emotionally and spiritually. After reading Sarah's story, I know it will encourage many to believe they too can heal from the inside out.

—**Tiffany Johnson,** Author, Speaker, Podcast Host, Screenwriter, Founder of When we are Brave

A courageous journey filled with a raw and pure vulnerability. *Infertility Saved My Life: Healing PCOS from the Inside Out* promises a rare insight into PCOS and infertility, the challenges, the triumphs and the wisdom gained. I confidently recommend this book to anyone who is walking a similar path.

—**Maria Lacey,** Registered Counsellor, Spiritual Mentor, Healer and Author

Sarah writes with a sensitive honesty that raises both tears and hope. In sharing her story we are invited to step alongside her, to understand and to learn and grow. Not just for those with fertility stories, *Infertility Saved My Life: Healing PCOS from the Inside Out,* shares a breadth of pragmatic skills to apply to every day life and the stresses it throws up.

—**Sarah Carroll,** Educator

Infertility
SAVED
MY LIFE

Healing PCOS *from the Inside Out*

Sarah
Willoughby

NEW YORK

LONDON • NASHVILLE • MELBOURNE • VANCOUVER

Infertility Saved My Life

Healing PCOS from the Inside Out

© 2023 Sarah Willoughby

Published in New York, New York, by Morgan James Publishing. Morgan James is a trademark of Morgan James, LLC. www.MorganJamesPublishing.com

Proudly distributed by Ingram Publisher Services.

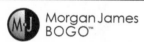

A **FREE** ebook edition is available for you or a friend with the purchase of this print book.

CLEARLY SIGN YOUR NAME ABOVE

Instructions to claim your free ebook edition:
1. Visit MorganJamesBOGO.com
2. Sign your name CLEARLY in the space above
3. Complete the form and submit a photo of this entire page
4. You or your friend can download the ebook to your preferred device

ISBN 9781631959097 paperback
ISBN 9781631959103 ebook
Library of Congress Control Number: 2022935285

Cover Design by:
Rachel Lopez
www.r2cdesign.com

Interior Design by:
Christopher Kirk
www.GFSstudio.com

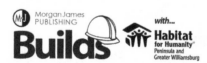

Morgan James is a proud partner of Habitat for Humanity Peninsula and Greater Williamsburg. Partners in building since 2006.

Get involved today! Visit MorganJamesPublishing.com/giving-back

Dedication

To every person who has experienced infertility, PCOS, miscarriage, and loss of a loved one, I believe you are stronger than you know. Never give up hope. You are not alone. May your toughest challenges become your biggest blessings.

To Isaac, Madison, and Grace, my three beautiful, amazing, and funny children: You are my greatest teachers. If not for you, this book would not exist. I love you beyond words. Thank you for your constant love, and for choosing me!

In memory of my grandpa, Charlie. Thank you for touching my heart. Just being in your presence made me feel calm, happy, and enough. Without even uttering a word, you ignited my curiosity about life beyond our physical existence, what connects us as humans, and our reason for being here. Your gift to me was inspiring me to seek my truth, be a better person, and to make a difference in this miraculous world.

You were right: "Nothing is ever as bad as it seems."

Contents

How to Use This Book

P art One of this book shares my life story and the heart-wrenching experiences I endured to welcome my three beautiful children into the world. You may wish to read this in one sitting or over several days.

In Part Two, you will find practical exercises and wisdom to support you to create a more positive relationship with Polycystic Ovary Syndrome (PCOS), infertility, and yourself. For me, the PCOS symptoms I experienced improved when I opened my heart and embraced this inner work. I therefore encourage you to dive in, and go on your own healing and awakening journey using the tools that changed my life. Dipping in and out of these chapters over a few weeks will give you time to process what comes up for you, reflect on the insights gleaned, and take positive action toward a more fulfilling future.

My deepest desire is that my story helps you heal and fall in love with yourself. I hope you discover magic in nature and feel supported by the Universe as you enjoy this wild ride called *life*. May you have the courage to pursue your dreams and find your truth, no matter what!

INTRODUCTION
Life Begins Right Now

Your soul has all the answers;
you just need to be brave enough to listen.

April 2009

"I want a cuddle, Mommy."

"I know, Isaac, I want to cuddle you too. But it hurts Mommy too much. I'm so sorry, darling."

Physically unable to reach my son's small body or hold him in my arms, I gently kissed three-year-old Isaac's cheek as he was carefully lifted close to my face. How I loved the feeling of his soft skin against my lips. I wanted to savor this moment forever.

Isaac's big, brown eyes looked deeply into mine. "We didn't get to see the giant teddy bear together. It's not far. Can we go now Mommy, please?"

"I so wanted to visit it with you, honey, but I can't move."

Fear flashed across Isaac's face as his eyes filled with tears.

"When I get better, Isaac, I promise I'll go to see the teddy. I'll take a photo and send it to you, okay?"

An eerie silence filled the hospital room as the enormity of what was happening began to sink in.

"Okay, Mommy. When are you coming home?"

"I'm not sure, darling. Soon, I hope. Be good for Grandma."

"I will."

"I love you, Isaac."

"I love you too, Mommy."

From my hospital bed, I watched my beautiful blond-haired son slowly walk out of the room. With tears in my eyes, I called out to him and mustered a smile. He waved his hand, clasping his well-loved jingling rabbit in the other. As the heavy, wooden door closed behind him, Isaac turned to look at me one last time, oblivious to the fact that we might not see each other again. And then he was gone.

Desperate to have a baby and repeatedly failed by the UK National Health Service (NHS), I had ventured to Norway to undertake an In Vitro Fertilization (IVF) cycle. IVF is a common procedure but it had unexpectedly threatened my life. Ovarian Hyperstimulation Syndrome (OHSS) struck me down with a vengeance. The fertility drugs caused my ovaries to seriously overreact, swelling to several times their normal size. Fluid rapidly leaked into my abdomen and lungs. My kidneys stopped working and my heart was enlarged. Powerless to stop the OHSS progressing, the doctors could only treat the symptoms as they presented themselves. I was not prepared for the trauma that occurred. I felt as though I was being tortured. My body battled to keep going as I faced the reality that I may not recover. Saying goodbye to Isaac was the hardest moment of my life.

The threat that my son could grow up without his mom weighed heavily on my mind. After he left, my heart pounded in my chest and I broke down in tears. Unable to breathe, the pain coursing through my body could no longer be contained. I was in agony. Morphine brought no relief. I was helpless, out of my depth, and after more than two years struggling with infertility, I wanted an end to it.

Years later, my soul still remembers that grueling time. During periods of reflection while lying in my hospital bed, I promised myself that if I recovered, I would wholeheartedly embrace each day and pursue a life of no regrets. My only remorse would be for those opportunities that I fearfully turned my back on and wasn't brave enough to try. With my body ballooned with fluid and my organs slowly shutting down, I prayed it wasn't too late.

***

Ever since I was seven years old, I have felt compelled to write. This feeling amplified in the years leading up to writing this book. It was as though something much bigger than myself, my soul, was calling me to put pen to paper. But I still wasn't sure exactly what I was supposed to express to the world. Eventually I surrendered. When I connected with my true essence and asked for clear guidance, the fog began to lift. This allowed my eyes to see, and my heart to feel the truth. Through this awakening, I discovered how unique we all are. I realized that my story about living with PCOS, my heartbreaking journey to be a mom, and the spiritual lessons that unfolded along the way could never be told by anyone else. This was the key to the next chapter in my life; it was time to stop hiding.

This book begins with me openly discussing my emotional challenges through puberty, diagnosis of PCOS, secondary infertility, miscarriages, IVF, and intensive care. I've also shared the tools and insight that helped me maneuver through the confusion of contradictory medical advice, drugs, and lack of support, to then manage PCOS and transform my whole life. I delve into the pain, loss, stress, and trauma I endured over thirty years, the spiritual transformation that entwined each experience, and the fascinating connection between our mind, body and spirit. The importance of opening your heart and mind to recognize who you really are and creating space to reconnect with your true desires through meditation, nature and mindfulness are covered. I also dive into the benefits of exploring creativity, journaling, intuition, vulnerability, mindset, love, fear, forgiveness, gratitude, grief, uncertainty, change, guilt, failure, and shame, so that despite the circumstances endured, you can still enjoy moments of joy. A toolbox and resources are shared to help you navigate through PCOS, infertility and miscarriage with more ease and grace. Lastly, there is a brief fact sheet about PCOS.

Today, I grasp that we are on a voyage back to self through our tribulations. This voyage is never-ending. Unarguably, we are at the mercy of this great adventure, with all its twists and turns, until we take our last breath. I aspire to lessen human suffering and provide a safe space for others to bravely walk toward their truth. Contributing to healing the planet motivates me to keep going, even when it feels uncomfortable. There is much to learn. Constantly seeking to be the best version of myself, sometimes I falter or make mistakes. That's okay. I don't always have the answers to my questions or know where I'll end up. I'm not meant to. But it doesn't mean I shouldn't begin. The same is true for you. I'm confident that if you allow yourself to embark on a self-discovery exploration, your spirit will awaken, your soul will be stirred, and life will begin to flow.

Despite feeling somewhat exposed while writing down my thoughts and feelings, I know that sharing my life with you is a necessary part of my healing. This book is dedicated to the millions of women (and men) all around the world affected by PCOS and infertility, who contend with the minefield of symptoms and obstacles that these conditions present. If my story inspires and empowers you to heal from the inside out and practice self-love, then my work is done. Life is short. Grab it with both hands, and make every moment count!

Part One

P art One of this book shares my deeply personal story. It's an honest and raw account about my life from puberty through to the birth of my third child. It wasn't always easy writing my thoughts down on paper, and there were many tears shed along the way. But whenever I considered giving up, I always received a divinely-timed message to persevere. I hope that as you read my story, you are inspired to keep going, talk about how you're feeling, and prioritize your well-being. I believe that when you're brave and express your vulnerabilities, you open the door to your own truth and healing.

CHAPTER 1

Puberty Blues

Tune into your body; ask questions and trust yourself.

I was born in England, in a historic market town called Pontefract in West Yorkshire, in 1978. My family was middle class, and I grew up with my mother, father and older sister. Winters were cold, dark, and snowy. The highlight of these dreary months was making snowmen with friends in the street outside our house.

Every June we retreated to France to camp, swim and enjoy the balmy summer evenings. When I was five years old, we moved down south to Cheltenham, a large spa town, in Gloucestershire. Most weekends were spent with my four grandparents exploring the charming, picturesque villages in the neighboring Cotswolds. My grandpa, Charlie, was particularly special to me. His big heart and warm smile always made me feel loved and safe.

The carefree moments of my childhood abruptly ended when I hit puberty. The whole affair daunted me. Not only was I battling the bewildering hormones most girls contend with when they start changing from a girl to a woman, but I was also dealing with PCOS. Not that I knew it. It took another thirteen years for this to be finally identified.

I had just turned twelve years old when my first period started. It was the summer holidays before I commenced my second year of secondary school. Leading up to my period's arrival, I had been quite keen for menstruation to start so I would fit in with those girls already ahead of me. But throughout the following months and years, I wished I could turn back the clock.

The day after my first period started, I took the train to London with my family for a long weekend. A visit to the big city was rare so I'd been looking forward to this mini adventure, but the sanitary pads I now needed to wear were thick and obtrusive. Like most teenage girls, I walked around convinced people could see them through my clothes. The thickness of the pads didn't match the protection they gave me. I was constantly anxious that I was going to leak all over my clothes and become a target for ridicule. Public toilets were scarce. Even going to a chemist with my mother to buy new sanitary pads was awkward. I felt ashamed that everyone would know what was happening to my body. The stomach cramps, backache, and seemingly never-ending bleeding also caught me off guard, making me miserable and out of sorts. For most of the trip, I longed to be at home tucked up in bed with a hot water bottle while I began to digest what was happening to me.

Between twelve and fourteen years old, I dealt with irregular menstrual cycles, agonizing uterine cramps, and excessive bleeding that made me run down and drained. Incessant backache meant I was not able to stand up for long, especially during days one and two of my cycle. Despite being prepared, and taking large supplies of sanitary products wherever I went, I was often caught out because I had no idea when my period would arrive or how long it would last. Accidents were frequent and embarrassing. Often menstruation would continue for up to twenty-one days. When it eventually stopped, I would breathe a sigh of relief, only for it to start all over again a few days later. Sometimes my periods were absent for six months, which was a welcome break, but then the next one invariably overcompensated for it.

Because it's common to have irregular cycles during the first one to two years of menstruation, diagnosing PCOS in young women is not straightforward. The many doctors I spoke to throughout the first few years all dismissed my erratic cycles and extensive bleeding as "normal" while my body settled down and went through the transition to becoming a woman. They explained it could take up to two years for my periods to become regular, less heavy and painful, and I lived with optimism that they were right.

Over the next few years, the pressure of attending a very academic selective school in the UK and all the extracurricular activities I was involved with rapidly increased. I was getting close to sitting my final exams, and I couldn't, and didn't, want to deal with the pain, exhaustion and unpredictability anymore. The wait-and-see game was proving to be a long one and there were no signs of improvement. Even though I remained hopeful that things would get better, when they didn't, I turned to alternative therapies. Reflexology helped to reduce tension in my body and bring calm to my mind. The reflexologist showed me which part of my hands and feet I needed to rub to alleviate pain in my uterus and ovaries, which fortunately made it more bearable.

Blood tests and a pelvic ultrasound would have clarified whether there were hormonal imbalances and follicles on my ovaries. Regrettably, these tests were never presented to me as options. A medical decision was made to put me on the pill at fourteen years old. I understand the strategy was to regulate my cycle and reduce my bleeding and pain so that I could live a more normal life. But now I know that the pill masked the full extent of the hormonal issues and imbalances my body was dealing with for another eleven years. The root cause of the problem was never located nor addressed. This scenario was akin to calling a plumber to fix a leaking pipe. Instead of investigating the real cause of the leak, rusting pipes, the plumber provided a temporary fix and tied an old rag around the hole. If the problem couldn't be seen, it didn't need fixing, right?

Wrong! It inevitably comes back to bite you on the bum, so to speak. For ten years, I took the pill, which helped regulate my cycle and prepared me somewhat for the hormonal avalanche each month. However, I was dosed up on painkillers just to function and my periods were relentless, particularly the first two or three days. Sometimes I would have to change a tampon, pad or both every couple of hours. As so many women do, I just got on with it, resigning myself to thinking I was unlucky, and that this was normal for me. I convinced myself that there was nothing else that could be done, which led to me presuming the problems were all in my head. Had I continued to ask questions and do more research, PCOS may have been identified sooner. I will never know. If I had my time again, I wouldn't have taken no for an answer. I would have stood up for myself, trusted myself more, and fought for my well-being. We live and learn!

CHAPTER 2

The Diagnosis and Living with PCOS

I am not crazy, but I am broken.

For a while being on the pill didn't cause too many unwanted side effects. It was certainly an improvement on what I had previously coped with, and I was appreciative of that. Fortunately, I've never had to deal with weight gain, excess body hair, acne, hair loss or glucose intolerance, which affects so many women with PCOS and causes a host of other problems. Nonetheless, when I left home at eighteen to go to university, the pill stopped working properly. Plymouth, a port city on the south coast of Devon, became my new home while I undertook a business studies degree and spread my wings. Visits to the doctor during my first year of studies became increasingly more frustrating and frequent.

"How can I help you today?" the doctor asked.

Feeling fed up, I replied, "I'm on Microgynon, but it's not working very well. My periods are heavy and I'm experiencing breakthrough bleeding."

"Have you missed taking any tablets?"

"No," I said.

I put across my concerns that there was more going on with my body that hadn't been investigated. The doctor listened but ignored my request to be referred to a specialist, suggesting my hormonal disruptions could simply be due to stress.

Putting my nagging doubts to one side, I conceded that maybe he was right, and I was worrying about nothing.

"Let's try a different type of pill. Another one may suit you better," he proposed.

As I took the prescription from the doctor's hand, I convinced myself that I just needed to be more positive and that this time would be different.

Over the next five years, I tried one brand of pill after another: Cilest, Logynon, Mercilon, Marvelon, the list went on. But each time, it would work for a while, until the side effects began to outweigh the benefits. The pill affected my mood, and the frequent spotting was getting worse. I felt like I was right back at the beginning. None of the numerous doctors I spoke to would refer me to the hospital for the necessary blood tests and ultrasound. By 2002, I could no longer put up with the hormonal changes and mood swings I had been experiencing for the past twelve years. Without consulting a doctor, for my mental well-being, I decided to come off the pill to give my body a break from the chemicals. For the first time in years, I felt more like me and wished I had been brave enough to do it sooner.

But, despite feeling much better within myself, something wasn't right. My period didn't start. Not the first month, nor the next month. It was over twelve months before my body naturally settled down. I knew stress wasn't the culprit either. I was now twenty-five, and I was no longer prepared to be fobbed off as I had been during my teenage years. Armed with this new information, at last, I came upon a doctor in 2003 who took me seriously.

"Have a seat, Sarah. How can I help?"

I was tired of repeating the same spiel, so, sensing defeat before I had even started to speak, I said, "When I was fourteen, the pill was prescribed. It worked reasonably well until I was about eighteen, but then the spotting became more frequent, and my periods intensified again. I tried different brands to find one that suited me. None of them worked, so almost twelve months ago I took myself off the pill. I've been better since, but I haven't had a period."

"Yes, your notes suggest you've been dealing with this for a while. I think it's time to refer you to a specialist."

"Really?" I asked with genuine surprise.

"Yes, I think it would be good for some further tests to be carried out. We've done everything we can here."

As the doctor typed up the referral letter, she confirmed that there would be at least a six-month wait for the hospital appointment under the NHS. These timescales were normal but longer than I had expected. Although disappointed, I was thankful that progress was at long last being made. My only other option was to pay for private medical appointments, which at the time I could not afford.

"Thank you," I said.

"You're welcome, Sarah. You don't have to suffer in silence. There are no prizes for being a hero! I hope you get some answers."

Appreciative that I was finally being taken seriously, I went home to tell my boyfriend, Giles, the good news. Giles and I had met when I was twenty years old, in 1998, during a placement in the third year of my business studies degree. This placement was spent working in the human resources (HR) department at Rolls-Royce in Bristol as an undergraduate trainee. Giles was an engineering graduate, and Friday nights were frequently spent socializing together in a large group of mutual friends. When I returned to Plymouth in 1999 to complete my fourth year of university, our friendship continued to blossom. In 2000, we began a long-distance relationship. Eight months later, once I had finished my final exams and traveled around Asia with a friend, I moved back to Bristol to be with Giles and pursue my HR career.

After many months of waiting for my hospital appointment, the day to speak to the specialist arrived. I was optimistic that an answer may be forthcoming, but at the same time, I was filled with dread in case it wasn't. The hospital waiting room was hot, small, and crammed full of other women all appearing equally anxious. I was a bag of nerves. Working in HR meant that I was constantly on call to deal with any staff issues that arose throughout the day. Conscious of being out of the office, I knew when I returned there'd be a mountain of files stacked on my desk, copious voicemail messages, and a ridiculous number of urgent emails in my inbox. I had decided not to book the day off as a holiday because I suspected I would need to have further medical tests and more time absent from work over the forthcoming months. Instead, I planned to make up the hours for this quick, routine appointment after 5:00 p.m.

The minutes ticked by. My nerves were now swirling around my stomach like an angry army of bees who'd had their nest disturbed. The anxiety heightened as I contemplated what was to come in the specialist's room, and later back in the office. After waiting for an hour, my name was finally called, and I followed the doctor into an uninviting consulting room. Question after question was fired at me and my complete medical history was written down in a bid to piece together my life over the past thirteen years. After a brief period of contemplation, the doctor advised me that when I was next bleeding, I would need to come back to the hospital for a blood test to check my hormone levels. Until then it was just a waiting game, and I knew it may be a long one. My heart dropped. This could be months. I left the hospital deflated. However, much to my surprise, I started menstruating later that day. I phoned the hospital and was able to book the relevant blood tests the following morning.

The day I returned to the hospital for my results, I was expecting to be told there was nothing wrong. I was mentally prepared to draw a blank, and concede that I needed to learn how to cope with the symptoms instead. After another long wait, a nurse with blonde, tightly curled hair and piercing blue eyes led me into a small, gloomy room. I sat down on the hard chair next to a wooden table, wishing I'd asked Giles to come to my appointment with me. The nurse flicked open my file and briefly scanned through my notes before casually stating:

"The blood tests show you have PCOS."

"Oh," I replied, gutted. One of my friends had been diagnosed with this some months prior. I knew she was feeling down about the diagnosis and agitated that her fertility could be compromised.

"Take the pill. There is no need for another appointment."

I paused for a second, trying to process what I'd just been told. Her lack of empathy had muted me.

"This can be dealt with through your doctor," the nurse tersely advised me.

I was angered by her impatience and need to get me out of the room as quickly as I had walked in.

"So, what about my fertility?" I asked. "I'm aware this can be affected. What do I need to know?"

"Nothing until you're ready to have a baby."

"I'm wanting to start a family in the next few years. I'm already twenty-five and would appreciate some information on PCOS. You haven't explained any-thing to me. Is there a leaflet I can have please?"

The words tumbled from my mouth and I burst into tears. Frustration had got the better of me.

Looking slightly taken aback, the nurse reached into a drawer and handed me a leaflet on PCOS. I thanked her and walked out of the hospital room, upset that there was no time to discuss what PCOS meant for me, how to manage my symptoms or where to get help.

Returning to work in a complete daze and unable to think, I sat at my desk. Fighting back the stream of tears, none of the HR issues that needed resolving seemed important. Work was the last place I wanted to be, and I couldn't have cared less about my job. I had so many unanswered questions and it felt like no one was listening or even cared. My chest tightened with anger as I suppressed an impulse to scream at the top of my lungs. All I wanted to do was fall into the safety of my bed and hide from PCOS and myself.

The day I was diagnosed with PCOS permanently changed my life. It was bittersweet. On the one hand, like so many other women, I was glad that PCOS had finally been identified. After years of asking doctors questions and searching for answers, I'd convinced myself I was either imagining the symptoms, stressed or simply had an overly active negative mind. I was thankful I wasn't crazy or delusional. On the other hand, I'd read that there was no cure for PCOS. I could only manage the symptoms. More crucially, I grasped that in the future, when I was ready to have a baby, PCOS could result in years of infertility, an increased risk of recurrent miscarriages and emotional torment. My heart cracked.

CHAPTER 3

Four Pregnancy Tests Later

Pregnancy glow. What's that?

G iles and I had been together for three years when I was diagnosed with PCOS. He wanted to start a family in the future, and I was keen for him to be the father of my children. But having researched what living with PCOS meant both in the short and long term, I was on tenterhooks that Giles would leave our relationship. I knew he loved me, but in spite of his reassurance to the contrary, I felt like damaged goods. Guilt set in. I feared I may not be able to give him the family he desired, and I was unsure whether he would stick around to find out.

Even though Giles listened with compassion to my concerns and reassured me, at times I still felt incredibly alone. Despite only being in my mid-twenties, in my head I was rapidly running out of time. I longed to start a family soon in case we struggled to conceive. Giles wanted to prioritize being able to financially provide for us, whereas I was driven by my hormones and the biological clock ticking loudly in my body. Some days it felt like a bomb ready to explode. My mind ran away with me and I fretted about things I had no control over. I didn't understand that this was a waste of energy and only made things worse. We attract what we focus on, and our mindset is pivotal to the experiences we have in life. Much later, I would learn this the hard way.

Exhausted from being unheard, I felt like nothing more than a chess piece that had been moved around a complicated and slow medical system. I was the problem that needed fixing, but there was no resolution in sight. I felt lost. Some days I coped better with this than others. I knew eventually I would have to lift my head out of the sand, face PCOS and the fears I was so deeply burying. But I wasn't ready. For the next few years, I rejected PCOS and blocked out how I felt by immersing myself in my career. I learned that society rewards busyness; busy equals important. Cramming my diary full of work obligations, I used my hectic schedule as an excuse to zone out of my personal life. With an overly analytical mind and a perfectionist streak, I was driven to achieve and succeed. I religiously followed the path that both I and others expected of me. I wasn't clear on my purpose, and lacked the insight that when we live with a more meaningful and deeper intention, hardships lessen and life flows.

At the time I didn't have the maturity, competence and strength to discern what would fill my heart, what I was passionate about. I did not understand that this was the key to a long and successful career in any chosen field. That doing more of what I loved would mean I had more to give, both professionally and personally. That passion would reenergize me and entice me to keep going, even when setbacks were encountered. As so many people do, I had entered the world of work with my head, not my heart.

Keen to progress in business, in 2002 I began a two-year postgraduate diploma in human resource management, while also working as a graduate. It was a good distraction, but I also knew this wasn't healthy. After I graduated in 2004, I recognized how overstretched I had been. But I kept going. My job became the center of my existence and I lived to work. The culture also recompensed presenteeism, not contribution. I began the year-long process to have my experience, skills and qualifications formally recognized by obtaining my chartered HR membership. I believed I would then have everything I needed, and the work pressure would subside.

But it didn't, and a real love-hate relationship with the very thing that occupied most of my thoughts and existence developed. My professional achievement was a major source of satisfaction, and brought meaning to my life. I loved helping people, encouraging them to resolve their problems, and picking them up when they fell. The roles I undertook were mentally stimulating, and the pay, benefits and job title were attractive. Money motivated me. I saw my income and personal possessions as a means of proving my relative worth compared to other people, as a status symbol. However, there was a darker side to the picture. The frustration of regularly having to put a band-aid on something, rather than getting to its root cause, slowly wore me down. Problem-solving focused on the short-term agenda, resulting in moving people along if they didn't quite "fit." I hated the bureaucracy and office politics and was not any good at it. The half-truths, game-playing and lack of integrity, as well as regularly being swamped by a never-ending workload, became increasingly stressful. Because I didn't have children, my managers and customers perceived my personal life to be less valuable. I was therefore expected to work regular overtime, even though my productivity was compromised. Often leaving the office exhausted, and feeling I hadn't achieved what I had planned to, I was conscious that more tasks would be waiting for me the next day. And then, of course, there were other urgent and unexpected issues to deal with each morning; ones I couldn't even prepare for. My resentment toward this perpetual cycle of pressure and intrusion into my personal life continued as I frequently completed work at night or on the weekend to ensure my career progression was not jeopardized.

As much as I was dissatisfied with my choice of profession, I believed that my six years already spent studying at university would be wasted if I changed careers. My ego stepped up to protect me and won the internal fight that took place in my mind. It convinced me I was too old to move backward and seemingly start again, and that it was too late to retrain. The irony of this is that I was still only twenty-six. I lacked the insight to know what I wanted to do instead, and so I remained stagnant. Being neurotic about taking the wrong turn and ending up in a similar situation later down the track led to indecision. Self-sabotage and fear kept me stuck in a job I was beginning to hate, for many years to come.

At least now that I had finished studying, Giles and I had more time to enjoy ourselves together at weekends. In May 2004, we visited Westonbirt Arboretum in the UK. Spring had arrived, and the air was filled with the subtle aroma of flowers. The sun warmed my face as we slowly wandered through the trees. Blissfully quiet, with only the distant sound of birds tweeting, Giles guided me to sit on a wooden bench at the end of an avenue of large trees. No one else was around.

As we sat next to each other, the silence relaxed me. I appreciated the solitude we had been granted, happy that it was just the two of us in our bubble of love. After about ten minutes, Giles reached into his pocket and slowly turned to face me.

As I looked into Giles's loving eyes, I heard the words, "Sarah, I was wondering if you would do me the honor of marrying me?"

Even though I had hoped a proposal would be forthcoming, I was still astounded now that it was here. My gaze was drawn to the sparkling diamond engagement ring Giles held out in front of me, and I gasped.

"Yes, you know I will," I laughed.

Giles breathed a sigh of relief and tenderly kissed me as he placed the engagement ring on my finger. I sat gazing at it through tears.

With wedding plans well underway, we also embarked on a much-needed six-week sabbatical from work beginning in December 2004. I had a passion for travel and was so excited when the day to set off on our escapade finally arrived. We visited friends in Hong Kong; the South Island of New Zealand; Sydney, Uluru, and Melbourne in Australia. I enjoyed my time in each place but fell completely in love with Melbourne the minute my feet touched the ground. Even though I had not been a fan of cities, the café culture, city trams and European vibe were appealing. An inner calmness touched my soul. I had never felt anything like it. Sensing I was home, I cried at the end of our trip as we prepared ourselves to return to the UK and the corporate rat race.

Back in the UK, my attention turned to our wedding plans. We married in May 2005 in a pretty, quaint church with stained-glass windows and an ornately decorated ceiling. Family and friends celebrated with us until the early hours of the morning with food, wine and a ceilidh that had all our guests dancing and laughing, particularly as the moves got more complicated and the dancing deteriorated. The same day we exchanged contracts on our new family home. Everything was falling into place.

We spent the weekend socializing with friends in the city of Newcastle before heading off on our honeymoon. Having already crossed Australia and New Zealand off our list, we decided to venture to Cape Town and Namibia in Southern Africa. We were blessed to see majestic wildlife, camp under the stars, skydive over the desert, and climb up massive sand dunes to watch the sunset. Barbecued meat by the fire at night was tender and flavorsome. I loved being outdoors. The entire trip resonated with my heart.

My twenty-seventh birthday was celebrated on safari with a chocolate cake from the local baker's, dancing, and one too many shots of Jägermeister. Woken early the following morning for our skydiving trip, I regretted the antics of the night before as my stomach turned inside out from both overindulging in alcohol and the anticipation of what lay ahead. Before I knew it, I was jumping out of the plane freefalling at high speed toward the ground. The exhilaration made me feel alive, and as my feet safely touched the warm earth, I smiled because my courage had been louder than my fear.

Out of all those wonderful memories, what I remember most is spending many hours peering out of the tour bus window, listening to Athlete's album on repeat. With the subtle tones of blue, green, pink and orange that effortlessly merged and intertwined, the landscape was like viewing one exquisite watercolor painting after another. The scenery was breathtaking, and it was one of the first times I had felt present in the moment and truly peaceful.

After our honeymoon ended, holiday blues kicked in. I became disillusioned at work and desperate to book our next trip away. Within a month, though, I started to feel nauseous. I thought a virus or work pressure had got the better of me. Even though I vomited throughout a whole day and night, I didn't seek medical advice, convincing myself I would recover in due course. On the 19th of July, 2005, after a few more days off work, I conceded and went to the doctor. We discussed all the symptoms, including aching breasts and the peculiar blue veins that were visible on my tender skin.

After a gentle examination, the doctor asked me, "Could you be pregnant?"

Bemused by the ridiculousness of the question, I laughed.

"Yes, in theory, I could be, but it's very unlikely. I have PCOS, am spotting, and haven't had a proper period for months. I don't even think I ovulate."

"Well, I would like to be sure." The doctor handed me a small plastic pot to provide a urine sample the next morning and return it to the surgery for pregnancy testing.

As I reluctantly left the doctor's room, I felt let down that I hadn't received any advice on how to feel better. Despite not using contraception on our honeymoon, I felt the test was a waste of time. After returning home, I curled up in bed with an overactive mind, feeling sorry for myself.

Since my PCOS diagnosis, I had wanted to protect myself from potential heartache, so I had mentally prepared myself for fertility issues. The suggestion that I could be pregnant therefore seemed ludicrous. In hindsight, bombarding my mind with negative thoughts about a situation that might not happen, and one that was out of my control, was particularly unhelpful. Tackling the problems only if they actually did arise would have been less emotionally draining, and better for my mental health. But at the time, unfortunately, I didn't have this insight.

As I lay in bed tossing and turning, I mulled over my conversation with the doctor. Convinced it would be nothing short of a miracle if I were pregnant, I wanted to rule this out before the idea drove me mad. Dragging myself out of bed, I walked into the local village and bought two pregnancy tests from the chemist. After returning home, I went straight upstairs to the bathroom and sat on the toilet reading the instructions on the packet; I had no idea what I was doing. Because I was tense and pressured, stage fright set in!

Normally I couldn't walk past a toilet without needing to go, so why was my body being uncooperative now? The test would be negative anyway. At last, I loosened up enough to wee on the stick. As I tentatively waited for the lines to become visible in the pregnancy test window, I noticed the dark blue paint beginning to peel off the bathroom walls. My hands trembled as I blinked to see the result. Then suddenly, there it was, without a shadow of a doubt. A plus appeared on the pregnancy test. I shook my head in disbelief. I couldn't be pregnant. This must be a mistake. Without thinking, I pulled out the second pregnancy test and repeated it. Moments later another cross appeared.

Even though I was clutching two positive pregnancy tests in my hands, I was still in complete denial. I washed my hands and ran downstairs, frantically tying up my shoelaces and grabbing my coat. Running into the village with my heart beating so fast I thought it may split open under the pressure, I returned to the same chemist and picked up two more pregnancy tests off the shelf. This time I chose different brands; I wanted to make sure I hadn't selected a faulty batch or taken the tests incorrectly.

Putting them carefully down on the counter, I complained to the lady behind the cash register how expensive they were.

"This will be the cheapest part of having a child," she chuckled.

"Yes, you're right," I laughed back.

That afternoon, £40 poorer and four positive pregnancy tests later, I was still skeptical that I was pregnant. Because I had expected conception to be problematic, I was astonished that it had all been so effortless. I phoned my sister-in-law for advice. She teased me, telling me I couldn't get a false positive unless I was taking drugs that could distort the results, which I wasn't, or had something wrong with me, which was unlikely. My spotting was implantation bleeding; I didn't even know this existed. A few days later, the doctor's urine test results came back positive. On reflection I was naive. Giles felt cheated that he hadn't got to enjoy the baby-making proceedings for longer but was delighted with the wonderful news.

My pregnancy was not an easy one. I bled on and off throughout the whole of the first trimester and was terrified I would lose my beautiful baby. My increased risk of miscarriage kept me on edge, and I felt as though my body, this PCOS body, was going to let me down again. I vomited all day, every day, and began to lose weight. On the 1st of August, 2005, at eight weeks pregnant, the doctor confirmed I was suffering from hyperemesis gravidarum (excessive morning sickness). During our discussion, he warned me that although it was exceptionally low risk, birth defects had been linked to anti-nausea medication. Desperate for some relief, I reluctantly took the doctor's prescription to the chemist and started taking the tablets. But I was riddled with guilt that I may be harming my growing baby. So when the excessive nausea and vomiting didn't ease, I stopped taking the tablets. Frequently running out of work meetings, vomiting in the car park or at the side of the road became part of my daily routine. This alien assault continued for seventeen weeks. I felt as though I was on a boat with the worst sea sickness imaginable and I couldn't get off. It exhausted me beyond comprehension. The only relief I got was during sleep. Upon waking, there was a blissful moment before nausea hit me again like a fierce wave crashing against the rocks.

It was impossible to keep my early pregnancy a secret, even if I'd wanted to. I begrudged anyone who dared to tell me about their pregnancy "glow". Nothing about me glowed. I also got fed up with well-intentioned people suggesting their sickness remedies, none of which worked, or worse still, telling me it was all just in my head. There were many occasions I wished the pregnancy would end so I could reclaim my body from the parasite that had invaded it. I felt deeply ashamed knowing that other women would do anything to swap places with me if it meant they could hold a baby in their arms nine months later. Until we have walked in someone else's shoes, we cannot fully appreciate what each of us endures.

During those awful months, the ultrasounds brought me comfort and joy. In July 2005, at my seven-week dating scan, I saw my baby's heartbeat for the first time. Though it didn't quite compute that the screen was showing my future son or daughter growing inside me, I loved the magic regardless. At my eleven-week scan, I was blessed to see and feel my baby kicking at the same time, like a butterfly fluttering inside me or a bubble slowly rising to the surface of the water and softly popping.

Everything started to seem real from this point onwards. With the risk of miscarriage now much lower, I was relieved when I reached the middle of the second trimester and my nausea and vomiting eased. Feeling like a new woman, I began to enjoy the pregnancy. With tremendous anticipation and excitement, I started counting down the months until I would meet my future child.

CHAPTER 4

The Birth of My First Child

Becoming a mom fills your heart with so much love and vulnerability. You don't know whether to laugh or cry.

F ast-forward to Christmas Day 2005, I was now six and a half months pregnant. After eating turkey and all the trimmings cooked by Giles, I stood at our lounge windows looking at the brightly colored cottages and church opposite. Smoke from the chimneys twisted and turned in the crisp winter sky, and I felt lucky to be living in such a beautiful village. Feeling tired, I curled up on the comfy sofa and fell asleep.

When I returned to work on the 2nd of January, 2006, I started to prepare the handover for my colleague who was going to be covering my maternity leave. Isaac was due on the 14th of March so I had planned to finish work in mid-February. I was looking forward to a break from my busy and stressful job. But I was not ignorant to the fact that soon motherhood would be the hardest challenge I had faced so far.

On Friday the 13th of January, 2006, a routine antenatal check with the midwife revealed my blood pressure was much higher than usual: 130/82. There was no other evidence of the serious condition, preeclampsia, except being tired, so the midwife wasn't too concerned at that stage. She advised me to go home and put my feet up over the weekend, which I did, and to return on Friday the 20th of January for another check-up.

Throughout the weekend, it became evident how lethargic I was. I had this nagging doubt, which I kept trying to ignore, that something wasn't quite right. I didn't get much sleep on Sunday night. For once I listened to what my body was telling me and the next morning called work advising them I was unwell. I'd had mild contractions since 3:00 a.m. but convinced myself they were just Braxton Hicks (practice contractions). Later that morning though, with a sickening sensation in the pit of my stomach, I plucked up the nerve to phone my midwife for reassurance. With tremoring fingers, I anxiously dialed the number, trying to slow down my breathing at the same time. My heart sank when I heard she was away from the office and my call was being transferred to a colleague who would be unfamiliar with my records.

"Hello, can I help?"

"Yes, I had an appointment on Friday. My blood pressure was higher than normal. I've been unwell all weekend, and I'm worried I'm having contractions."

The midwife listened to my concerns as I explained that I had been experiencing regular pangs for the past eight hours, even though I'd rested all weekend.

"Was your urine test normal and how many weeks are you?"

"Yes, it was normal," I replied. "I'm thirty-two weeks."

"You don't seem to be in too much pain," she retorted. "As you're only thirty-two weeks, it's likely to be Braxton Hicks. But if you are concerned, I suggest going to the hospital to be checked."

Feeling dismissed, the conversation ended without me receiving the reassurance I desperately needed. Convinced it must all be in my head, I returned to bed, scolding myself for phoning in the first place.

At 6:00 p.m. that evening, our financial adviser arrived. Unable to concentrate on the discussion, I listened to the regular chiming of the church bells. The sound usually warmed my heart, but today, the same bells confirmed that my contractions were now fifteen minutes apart. My disquiet returned and remained with me all night.

It was now around 10:00 a.m. on Tuesday the 17th of January. Still not well enough to return to work, I stayed in bed and tried to keep warm. Drifting in and out of sleep, I was woken by an unexpected but welcome call from my midwife, Mary. It was good to speak to someone who knew me and my medical history; she seemed to take my concerns more seriously. After about five minutes, Mary calmly advised me to pack a bag and go to the hospital, reassuring me that it was just a precautionary measure. I phoned my husband with the update, and he gathered up his belongings and returned home. Neither of us perceived how serious it was. We both thought the baby may just be lying in an awkward position, and the false alarm would mean Giles could return to work after lunch.

The midwife rang the hospital and advised them I would be arriving shortly. As I walked into the surprisingly silent birthing suite reception at 11:30 a.m., I had no idea where anything was or what to expect; my hospital tour was in four days. We were greeted by a pretty, young midwife with long, curly hair. Smiling sweetly, she intently scanned my body and listened to how I spoke. I knew she was establishing if I was an attention-seeking fraud, panicked first-time mother or indeed in the early stages of labor. After a few moments, she concluded that I was probably not in labor because I was able to walk. Shame flashed across my face, so bothered was I that I was about to steal a midwife's valuable time from another woman who truly needed her.

"Come with me," the midwife gestured.

Like a naughty child who was about to be exposed for lying, I followed the midwife to a small, chilly area of the hospital with a low, camp-style bed hidden behind a thin curtain.

"Please undo your shirt and lie down," the midwife requested.

I wanted to apologize and say I was mistaken. That I was happy to go home and continue resting, and that I was sure it would pass. But no words came out. I tentatively lowered myself onto the small bed, thankful that I didn't crumble in a heap. An electronic sensor was placed on my tummy to measure potential contractions. Firmly held in place by an elastic belt, the sensor was attached to a wire which was connected to a machine. Another sensor was put over my baby's heart to measure their heartbeat, and the machine was set to work. With each tightening of my stomach, I watched the machine busily recording its findings. After about thirty minutes, much to everyone's surprise, the truth was revealed. My twinges were unequivocally real contractions; my midwife had been right to send me to hospital.

An uncomfortable, internal examination followed, confirming that my cervix had started dilating; I was in labor. Happy to neither be a fraud nor a panic-stricken first-time mother, my ego was rapidly tamed by the realization that I was not ready to meet my baby. Not on these terms anyhow. Even though I had read that women with PCOS are at an increased risk of delivering a premature baby[1], I hadn't considered this could happen to me. The mood of the midwives changed. They became more serious and focused on preventing my labor from progressing. This thirty-two-week-old baby was not to be born now; it was too early. A needle was briskly inserted into the back of my hand. An intravenous (IV) drip began pumping strong medication into my body to stop my contractions.

Despite receiving regular reassurance from the doctors and midwives that the drugs were likely to take effect and I would be sent home soon to rest, my gut instinct did not agree. PCOS was loudly stamping its feet again and interfering with my life; I couldn't escape it. I was concerned that I hadn't attended any "how to give birth" antenatal classes and aggrieved that I may not be able to enjoy my maternity leave and rest my body before I became a mom. *Will I have a premature baby? This can't be happening.*

Time ticked by and I reminded myself that this internal dialogue was not helpful. I made a conscious decision to try to push through my fears. Positive thinking would turn the situation around. I was managing the pain well, and there was still time for the contractions to stop. Or so I thought.

A few hours later, when it became clear that the medical team was less certain of the outcome, I was transferred to one of the empty birthing suites. The room was hot, but it felt cold and sterile with all the machines, monitors, and basic furniture. I hated hospitals; they filled me with dread.

When I was only two years old, I was admitted to the hospital with a nasty virus. My sister had been rushed into the same hospital the day before in an ambulance. As I kicked and screamed, afraid and in pain, a doctor and nurse tried to give me an injection in my arm. When I wouldn't cooperate, they asked my mother to leave the room before pinning me down to get the job done. That vivid scene feels like yesterday.

The birthing suite was larger than I expected–the reason for this would become apparent in due course. I appreciated the seclusion it granted me, but my mobility was relatively limited, and soon I was sore from lying down for so long. I waited. There was still the likelihood that my contractions would stop of their own accord and everything would be fine. But as the hours ticked by, one of the midwives became increasingly concerned that my contractions were coming closer together. No internal vaginal examination had been carried out by a doctor since I had arrived at the hospital almost twelve hours earlier. The pain was increasing. She was convinced I would be giving birth shortly. I was not ready, and neither was Giles.

At 8:30 p.m., the midwife decided to call the Neonatal Intensive Care Unit (NICU) so they could explain what would happen if our baby was born early. An Indian lady with a warm demeanor came into my room. I liked her instantly. With her, she brought an incubator, the place our baby would call home for the foreseeable future. When she explained to us that our baby would be connected to all sorts of wires and monitors, and need help breathing, it finally hit me. *This is not what I want. Will my baby be okay? It's too soon for both of us.* As she talked, I tried to suppress the panic rising through my tense body.

"When you're in the advanced stages of labor, the NICU team will be called. You won't be allowed to give birth until two pediatric doctors are present. Unless an obstetrician has to be paged, the midwives will deliver your baby and then hand them straight over to the NICU team to be checked and for help breathing. The room will be busy," she said.

Of course the room needs to be spacious.

"Will I be able to hold my baby?"

"No, sorry. Your baby will need to be placed straight in the incubator after the initial tests and taken straight to intensive care."

"Oh."

"Your baby will be very small when it's born, less than 4.5 pounds, and is unlikely to be able to breathe alone. They must get help immediately."

As she showed me the rough size of my baby with her hands, my heart lurched.

"How long will my baby need to stay in hospital?"

"Two months," she replied. "Babies born at thirty-two weeks tend to do quite well, but there are no guarantees."

I couldn't get these last words out of my mind. I was devastated that my baby would be rushed away before we had even been able to say hello or kiss their face. There would be no skin-to-skin contact, first feeds or happy family photos. Rather, a potentially strained, chaotic delivery that would pass us by in a blur. Giles was quiet, taking everything in that we had just been told. Neither of us spoke.

The doctors had tried to interfere with me as little as possible. But at 9:20 p.m., the midwife's persistence paid off and another internal check was reluctantly performed. Much to everyone's dismay, my body had fought gallantly against the drugs and the battle was over. My cervix was now 2 centimeters dilated, and there was no chance of stopping the labor. The doctors conceded, ceased all the drugs and advised me I was going to have this baby in the morning, eight weeks early.

Apprehension and unease took over my mind. *How will I get through the delivery?* I hadn't learned about the different stages of labor. I didn't know what to expect. Giles had no idea how to support me. Hearing the news that my baby could be sick or not survive after they were born was too much. *No! Stop this!*

Physically, I was unprepared to give birth. Random berating and trivial thoughts kept popping into my head as the adrenalin surged through my fatigued body. *Oh no, I haven't shaved my legs for a few weeks. The midwives are going to have to touch my prickly legs. How embarrassing.* Though it didn't matter, this is what was swirling through my crazed mind. As I lay in the hospital bed whiling away the hours, I desperately tried to push aside my concerns that I was not ready to become a mom tomorrow. It appeared I had no choice.

My husband phoned both our mothers. When Giles confirmed that the birth of our first baby was imminent, he was greeted by long silences. Up until now, he'd managed to remain calm, perhaps presuming it would never get to this point. But the seriousness sunk in once Giles said the words, "Sarah's in labor. The doctors have told us she'll have the baby in the morning. They can't confirm everything will be okay. I thought you should know."

Around 11:00 p.m., the midwives sent Giles home to get some sleep and advised us they would call him in the morning when it was time to come back to the hospital for the birth. As I tossed and turned in bed, loneliness and fear set in. I searched inside myself and asked for courage to get through whatever lay ahead. My grandpa was also at the forefront of my mind. I still missed him terribly. He died when I was only thirteen. My love for him was immense. He'd been such a positive role model and a fundamental part of my childhood. What I wouldn't do to have one more moment with my grandpa. I asked him to look after us both and keep my baby safe. An instant calmness washed over me as I felt his strong presence. My mind and body relaxed, surrendering to all that was meant to be.

Steroids were administered at 1:30 a.m. to help my baby's lungs and brain develop faster and reduce the risk of serious complications or death. Now there was nothing more the doctors could do except let nature take its course. Even though I was apprehensive about what was to come, I also believed we were protected. I knew my baby's life was in the hands of a power greater than me; all I could do was breathe through my fear and trust all would be well.

At 6:45 a.m. another internal examination revealed that my cervix was now 6 centimeters dilated. My contractions were intense and frequent. The midwife phoned my husband at 6:50 a.m. to advise him to come back to the hospital. When Giles entered the room, I felt relieved that he had made it in time, and I felt more confident with him by my side. As I prepared for our baby to enter the world, I put my faith in the Universe; there was nothing more I could do.

By 9:45 a.m. my cervix was fully dilated, and I was desperate to push. The pediatrician received an urgent call to attend and arrived in the birthing suite five minutes later with a colleague. At the exact time my antenatal class were gathered learning how to give birth, I was doing it for real.

The midwives supported and reassured me during each stage of labor and, somehow, I managed to keep myself together. Giles offered tender words of encouragement, sensing I was beginning to doubt whether I had the strength to do this.

Our baby was born at 10:32 a.m. in a room full of people. Waiting to hear the first cry felt like an eternity. Every second felt like a minute and every minute like an hour. My heart began to pound as I panicked. *Is something seriously wrong with our baby? Have I given birth to a boy or a girl?* I was too frightened to ask.

At the same time, I was relieved I had got through it and the contractions had now stopped, although the after pains were still unpleasant. The umbilical cord was cut, and the pediatric team whisked our baby off to the other side of the room to provide oxygen and carry out their checks. No one was talking. Silence filled the room, which seemed to have dropped a degree in temperature. Giles and I looked at each other, our eyes questioning why our baby had still not cried. I looked down and became aware of my deflated, saggy stomach and my sweaty, smelly body. I was exposed and vulnerable. Many more moments passed before an audible cry could be heard, a sound that brought tears of joy to my eyes.

"Congratulations, you've had a boy!" one of the midwives announced, as she placed her hand lightly on my shoulder. I looked up and smiled. Among all the chaos, they'd forgotten to tell me.

"Your baby's a good weight for thirty-two weeks," confirmed the pediatrician. "He weighs 4 pounds 6.5 ounces."

"Have you thought of a name for your son?" the second midwife asked.

"Isaac," I said beaming. In Hebrew, Isaac means "He will laugh; he will rejoice." Gratitude flooded from my heart. I was a mom.

Because the initial health checks indicated that Isaac was doing quite well, I was permitted to cuddle him briefly before he was placed in the incubator. As I held Isaac's tiny body in my arms, he looked back at me with his deep blue eyes and I fell hopelessly in love with him. The bond was instant; he was perfect. A quick blurry photo was snapped of us all together, then Isaac was taken away to receive oxygen.

I watched my newborn son's delicate body being placed in his incubator and wheeled out of the door to NICU for further testing. A wave of sadness surged through my body; this was not how it was meant to be. Giles wasn't allowed to hold Isaac in the delivery suite and still remembers the detachment he felt until he did. Those first brief moments were gone in an instant, never to be relived or reclaimed. All these years later, I'm still sad that we missed this special time together as a new family.

With no time to dwell on this, my attention was quickly pulled back to the room. I delivered the placenta, and the doctor sutured up the second-degree tears in my perineum. Neither was pleasant. After finishing my tea and toast, the midwives prompted me to have a bath, my first in three days. I needed to wash off the evidence of childbirth and change into clean clothes. The volume of blood that gushed out of my body onto the bathroom floor caught me off guard. This was another harsh reminder about how mentally unprepared I had been for Isaac's birth.

As I lowered myself into the water, I was in shock that I was now a mom. I was exceptionally sore and had a stretched stomach that no longer had a baby in it. As I sat in the bath, the midwife knelt beside the bath and softly washed my hair with all the tenderness you would treat a sick child. I recall the warm water pouring over my back. Resisting the tears of appreciation, relief flooded my body.

CHAPTER 5

Life in NICU

*Nothing can prepare you for that moment
when you must surrender to a power greater
than yourself and trust all will be well.*

After I had finished my bath, I was advised that we could visit Isaac.
My stomach swirled with nervous excitement; I suspected I'd burst into tears the moment I saw him.

As we negotiated our way through the never-ending hospital corridors, I was glad I had accepted the midwife's offer of going to NICU in a wheelchair. Until now I hadn't appreciated how worn out my body was or how much it had been through in the past forty-eight hours. The whole neonatal department was well protected with extensive security measures to keep the susceptible babies safe. Cameras and locked doors prevented anybody except the parents and medical teams from entering. Before being buzzed in by a member of staff, it was paramount to apply antibacterial hand sanitizer to reduce the risk of infection.

At the end of yet another long corridor, my heart pounded so loudly in my chest I thought someone else might be able to hear it.

"Are you ready?" the midwife asked us both.

"As ready as we'll ever be," I replied with an apprehensive laugh.

We reapplied more hand gel at the door and cautiously entered the room. It looked like an aquarium. The fifteen glass tanks scattered around the room were not filled with pretty, colored fish. Instead, each tank was home to someone's sick child, a baby battling to survive.

Machines beeped, alarms rang, monitors flashed.

One of the nurses came over to us and checked our parents' badges. She guided us to Isaac's incubator which was in the middle of the room. I breathed out, unaware I'd been holding my breath.

Scanning the room, panic rose in my chest as we walked closer to Isaac. There was nowhere to hide my emotions. Every direction I turned, other parents closely watched me with a sad curiosity. No one spoke or smiled; they were lost in their hurt. This silent, lonely place horrified me. I didn't want to be here; I didn't want my baby to be here.

"Isaac's just here," the nurse said, smiling. "You can stay as long as you'd like to."

As I saw my son for the first time, my stomach tightened into a stiff knot. Nothing could have prepared me for this moment. All alone in his incubator, Isaac's minuscule, naked body looked frail. He lay flat on his tummy, a crisp white sheet covering the thin mattress. Isaac's delicate feet touched a rolled-up, yellow knitted blanket that had been placed around the bottom half of his body, like a nest. He wore the smallest white nappy I had ever seen, and a white hat covered his soft dark hair to protect him from the cold. One thumb curled around a splint that was attached to Isaac's right forearm, preventing him from pulling out the sharp needle inserted into the back of his hand. A clear oxygen mask with gray elastic straps covered his face and a plastic feeding tube had been inserted into Isaac's stomach through his mouth. I hated all the machines and tubes, but I knew these were keeping him alive.

"Oh Isaac, I'm so sorry," I gasped.

Unable to sustain Isaac full term, I had failed him. Now his first few months of life would be spent in the hospital.

"This doesn't feel real," I whispered to Giles.

"I know," Giles replied with sorrow in his voice. "He doesn't feel like my son."

The disconnection washed over me like a wave. Guilty, I stared at Isaac curled up alone in his plastic box. His box of hope. The irony of listening to Athlete's song "Wires" countless times on my honeymoon in Namibia, now played out. I never thought I would relate to the lyrics as I did now. Examining Isaac, he had so many wires going into his body and coming out of his skin. My tears were driven by fear. *What happens if Isaac doesn't make it?*

Unsure how much longer I was going to be able to keep myself together, I noticed Giles was also grappling to do the same.

"I just want to touch him. I can't even stroke his hand," I said. Looking at me through the incubator, Giles nodded with tears in his eyes.

Panic flooded my mind as a mixture of adrenalin and sadness pumped through my weary body. Wondering whether it would be safer to emotionally detach from Isaac to protect my battered heart, I was terrified that he was going to be taken from me. That he was only supposed to be with us for the shortest time.

"Would you like to sit down?" One of the nurses gestured to the chairs she'd brought over for us.

Sitting in the chair, I became aware of subdued conversations between doctors and parents. The room lacked privacy; it had no screens or quiet corners to snuggle your baby, cry or just rest, away from prying eyes. Nurses moved from one incubator to another caring for each baby, readjusting tubes, oxygen masks, monitors and machines. I observed how vastly different the babies were both in size and age, wondering about their stories as they patiently waited for their next visitor. Even though we knew we could sit by Isaac's incubator and watch him sleep for as long as we wished, exhaustion crept up on me and we left NICU after an hour so I could rest.

There was much more I was unprepared for. While my husband drove home to get me some clean clothes and toiletries, I was transferred to the busy maternity ward. Walking into the room, I could see four beds. Mine was next to the large double doors which were propped open to the noisy corridor abuzz with a flurry of medical staff. Instantly hit by a wave of heat and pain, the medication was wearing off and I became aware I had lost all sense of time. I tentatively lay on top of the bed, thankful to be able to rest for the first time in days. Flowers, balloons and laughter filled the room. The three other smiling mothers were cradling their babies with love and tenderness. Surrounded by their happy families, celebrations were in full swing as the newest additions to each family were welcomed into the world. Wincing in pain with every small movement, I pushed myself up off the bed and slowly drew the curtains before lying back down again.

This was not my story. Clenching my stomach as though I'd been punched hard, the separation impaled me. Sick with worry, I watched the most pertinent chapter of my life play out from the sidelines. Desperate to get some much-needed sleep and block everything out while Giles was at home, I turned onto my side and closed my eyes. But I couldn't sleep, my mind was agitated.

Later that afternoon, at 3:45 p.m., one of the midwives unexpectedly approached me.

"We need you to change beds so a mother and her baby can move into this room. The one she's in is not warm enough for her baby."

"Oh," I replied with surprise. "When are they arriving?"

"Now."

I sat up and began to gather my limited belongings. Even though I understood the reasons I had been asked to move, and was happy to do so to help another new mother, inside I was silently screaming. The midwife's request was reasonable, but her delivery had been insensitive, and I was already sensitive enough. All I had wanted was for someone, anyone, to ask me how Isaac and I were doing or if I needed anything. It felt as though the absence of my baby was being ignored, and I was just another number on the production line.

I awkwardly shuffled into the noticeably chillier room; it was still tender to walk. As before, there were four beds, all unoccupied. I hoped this would remain the case so I could rest and mull over what was happening. Shortly after I moved rooms, one of the midwives gave me a digital photograph of Isaac. She advised me it would help with bonding and expressing milk for him, which was something I needed to start doing straight away. I thanked her and smiled, but as I looked at the baby in the photo, I didn't recognize him as mine. *Has there been a mix-up?* He looked completely different from the baby I had briefly held some hours before.

At 5:00 p.m., even though I'd asked to sleep for a while to recover from my ordeal, I was abruptly woken by one of the midwives to express milk. The sooner I could provide this for Isaac the better it would be for his health and development, and I was keen to cooperate. This first attempt was painful, embarrassing, and demoralizing. I was told to remove my top and undo my bra, before being handed a small syringe and shown how to squeeze my breast with my hand. No matter how much I tried, nothing came out because my milk hadn't come in yet. The midwife took over and persisted with her firm hands and fierce determination for at least another twenty minutes. She only managed to express 0.05 milliliters of colostrum from each breast; I felt like I had let Isaac down. Thankful when the midwife finally gave up and left, I turned over to cry.

When Giles returned to the hospital, I felt great comfort. He was the only other person who understood what I'd been through over the past forty-eight hours. Being with him helped to reduce some of the loneliness and frustration I'd been experiencing. At 7:15 p.m., we went back to NICU together to look through the incubator at our son. While I was silently pleading that all would be well, I heard a voice saying:

"Hello, I'm one of the pediatric doctors looking after Isaac."

"Hi," I replied, "How's he doing?"

"The test results when he was born were quite positive. We need to check whether there's bleeding on the brain, among other things. The results should be back within twenty-four hours."

I couldn't bring myself to question what would happen if the results were not favorable. The doctor's calm and warm demeanor helped me relax as he reassured us they were doing all they could.

"Thank you," I said.

"You're welcome. Would you like to hold your son?"

"Sorry?" I stuttered.

"If you'd like to hold Isaac, just ask the nurse to help you when she's finished with the other baby."

Giles and I both hesitated. Terrified that we would hurt our premature baby, we vigorously reapplied the hand sanitizer and sat down with anticipation, our trepidation rapidly turning to excitement. The nurse suggested I unbutton my shirt to enable skin-to-skin contact. When she placed Isaac's minute body on my bare chest, I felt his warm breath on my neck and his heart rising and falling against mine.

"Hello Isaac, I'm your mom," I whispered through a veil of tears.

My heart melted all over again. I didn't ever want to let him go. After what felt like only seconds, I realized I needed to give Giles the chance to hold his son for the first time. Conscious of all the wires, we were scared about accidentally pulling them, and inadvertently setting off the noisy machines. We called the nurse for help, who carefully passed Isaac over to Giles.

Isaac looked even tinier in my husband's arms. My heart filled with love for the second time that evening. With tears in his eyes, Giles smiled down at Isaac and tenderly kissed the top of his head. Special moments like these kept me going, helping me to get through the turbulent highs and lows of NICU life. Glancing around the room at all the sicker babies in their incubators, as we got up to leave I knew we had a lot to be thankful for. Isaac stood a fighting chance.

We returned to the draughty maternity ward which reminded me that it was the middle of winter, and Giles left soon after. At 9:00 p.m., I was instructed to express by hand again; I was too drained to protest. This time 0.16 milliliters of colostrum was collected, which was an improvement. I longed to be left alone to get some proper rest.

I was shattered, but couldn't get the sleep my body and mind pleaded for. Firstly, I was battling with my fear of hospitals. Since my traumatic childhood experience, I had only been in a hospital when somebody I loved was dying. Secondly, lying in bed without my son was soul-destroying. Thankfully, at long last, I drifted off to sleep around midnight.

"Argh!" A loud, high-pitched scream woke me with a start.

Through the smog of exhaustion and medication, I tried to make sense of what was happening.

Nurses were restraining a lady in the bed opposite as she writhed around.

"We're here to help you," one of the nurses said. "Stop kicking us. You need to calm down so we can give you some pain relief."

After an hour, the sorrowful groans and sobs lessened. I closed my tired eyes, determined to get some much-needed sleep. One of the midwives had promised I would be left alone until morning.

Yet shortly afterwards, around 3:00 a.m., I was woken again by a grumpy, close-to-retirement midwife who did not appear to enjoy her job.

"Up you get, Sarah–you need to express more colostrum for Isaac."

Half asleep and confused, I was left in the chilly, dark room with a tiny syringe and told to squeeze my breasts and nipples until I collected more drops of liquid gold. Unable to properly see what I was doing, unsurprisingly this method was ineffective. I had let Isaac down yet again. Reluctantly, I rang my bell for help.

"I'm struggling. Please can you help me?"

"What's the problem?" the intolerant midwife asked.

"I've been trying for twenty minutes, but it's not working," I warily admitted.

The midwife sighed, firmly squeezing my left breast and nipple. Her touch was rough and impatient. She continued for fifteen minutes before moving to the other side.

"Ow," I squirmed.

"I know it hurts, but your son needs this."

I wished the midwife would give up, but she seemed to be on a mission. I was sore and humiliated. However, the midwife carried on poking and prodding me for another ten minutes like I was a cow needing to be milked. Two or three drops of colostrum later, she got up to leave, saying:

"Your milk production must be stimulated; you'll be woken every two hours."

Disheartened, I rolled over crying, desperate for morning to arrive.

At 6:00 a.m. I awoke to the sound of staff chatting as they went about their early morning duties on the ward. Aware that my breasts were like rocks, and sore, I looked down and touched them. They had grown almost three cup sizes overnight! No wonder I was in agony. They felt like they didn't belong to me and I wondered how I'd manage to squeeze them into my bra.

I was instructed to express again at 7:00 a.m. and immediately became disgruntled. Thirsty, hungry and overly tired, I only managed to obtain a few drops. *When would this never-ending activity ever stop?*

An hour later, at breakfast, one of the midwives sat down on my bed. "I'm sorry you were woken in the night. You shouldn't have been. It was in your hospital notes to leave you to sleep but the night shift midwife ignored this."

"Yes, it would have been good to get some rest."

"It was too soon for your milk to have come in and your body needed time to recover from the birth. You've been through a lot," she said.

"I felt like such a failure last night," I replied. "Thank you for talking with me; I appreciate it."

The conversation ended and I turned my attention to getting dressed and organized for the day ahead. Shortly after breakfast, I was told that my bed was needed by someone else, and it was time to leave the hospital. It was still only 9:30 a.m., less than twenty-four hours after I had given birth.

I was glad to be going home with Giles, though it felt wrong for us to be walking out of the hospital doors without our baby. This was not how I had pictured it. In the car, my body hurt all over as though it had been in a ferocious war. My empty, sore tummy ached for Isaac as I thought of him alone in his plastic box. When I walked inside our house, I sighed. I may get some rest, but the place felt lifeless without the cries of my newborn son.

Returning to the hospital later that day to see Isaac, I was shown how to use the hospital breast pump, which was in a poky, communal room. I hated the pump. It was brutal, painful and unnatural. The pressure from the doctors and nurses to express was immense, and my body was not cooperating. Some women came into the room and sat jabbering with their friends or family while they expressed, as though it was the most natural thing ever. I preferred not to have an audience. While I was embarrassed that my milk was not in and I was barely expressing anything, they, on the other hand, collected enough milk to feed quintuplets. I convinced myself that it would be easier to express at home, where I could relax, and decided to invest in a breast pump.

Such is life with a premature baby–I needed to express milk around the clock. The first night, in the middle of a freezing January, I ran a warm bath and tried to express some more milk. The hot water was supposed to relax me as well as stimulate milk production, both of which I desperately needed. It was still excruciating. Despite the gut-wrenching cold and shooting pains, I kept going. No luck.

Setting my alarm for two hours later, I repeated the same exercise over and over until it merely became that thing I did, anytime, anyplace, and anyhow. Expressing milk was not going to defeat me.

Visiting Isaac in the hospital every day was tough. We faced minor gripes such as a lack of parking, a long walk into the hospital, limited room to sit next to the incubator, no privacy, and sore hands from the frequent reapplication of the abrasive gel. No amount of moisturizer seemed to reduce the rawness, and this was a constant reminder of what was happening in the hospital, even when I wasn't there. The nurses were pleasant enough, but for their sanity and profession-alism they were understandably detached from our situation. Some joked that we should make the most of the time to rest, and the free babysitters, because soon I would be up feeding throughout the night. But all I longed for was to have Isaac home with me.

Five days after our son was born, Giles had to attend a course in Edinburgh, Scotland. He was studying for a postgraduate diploma. If he hadn't gone, he would have had to wait another twelve months or longer to complete this part of the course, which neither of us wanted. Isaac's initial test results had been rela-tively reassuring. There was nothing Giles could physically do while he was in the hospital, except be patient and see how Isaac responded. But when Giles left for Scotland, copious tears engulfed me. My perineum was still healing and I could barely sit down, so driving myself to the hospital was exceptionally uncomfort-able. The hospital visits were lonely without Giles by my side. I missed his sup-port, which was vital so I could focus on my recovery and produce much-needed sustenance for Isaac. The saddest day was when Isaac was reweighed.

"Take Isaac's clothes off, but leave his nappy on until the last minute," said the nurse.

I reached inside the incubator. Undoing the poppers on his blue sleepsuit, I gently pulled Isaac's arms and legs out, trying not to hurt him. I carefully lifted his head to take off his bodysuit. Isaac's tiny body was warm. It was covered in lanugo, a fine fuzz that was soft to the touch. I hated disturbing him.

"When you're ready, remove Isaac's nappy and we'll weigh him," the nurse said, smiling.

Placing him on the metal scales, I watched as the number settled.

"Is that normal?" I said.

"Weight loss is normal for all newborns," the nurse reassured me, "but it's more than we would like."

Isaac now sat well under 4 pounds. My breast milk couldn't have been provid-ing the nutrition he desperately needed to put on weight, and gather the strength to suck and feed properly. The longer it took for Isaac to achieve both, the longer he would be stuck in the hospital where he was at risk of contracting an infection that could compromise his well-being, and set him back even further.

Desperate to take Isaac home as soon as I could, this latest news was not well received by me. After I left the hospital, I phoned my friend and cried. I wasn't used to being this vulnerable; I was ashamed that I wasn't coping. Despite her reassurance that all would be okay, that night I went to bed alone and frightened.

The prospect of holding Isaac close and smelling his soft skin against my body each morning always filled me with great anticipation and joy. Isaac opened his eyes and tried to look at me whenever he heard my voice saying his name. Sitting in the hospital for hours, as Isaac nestled on my chest fast asleep, became my daily ritual. The room was stifling. At times it was impossible not to fall asleep, although it helped that the chairs were rigid. Parents, nurses, doctors and specialists milled in and out of the small room to the backdrop of beeping machines. I saw many anxious parents settling in new babies, and tearful goodbyes for the families who were finally discharged.

I cared for Isaac as much as I could. Cotton wool balls soaked in warm water were used to clean Isaac's soft face and body before changing his little nappy. The Sterifeed plastic bottle containing my breast milk was warmed up on a radiator every four hours, before putting it into the thin tube inserted through Isaac's mouth to his stomach. One day a young nurse came to speak to me.

"I'm sorry, I accidentally spilled a bottle of your expressed milk as I took it out of the fridge."

I looked at her and tried to smile. "That's okay."

She walked off and I sighed with frustration. Even though it was an honest mistake, I knew she could not fathom how much effort, time and despair had gone into producing such a small amount of milk. Tears ran down my face as I took myself back to the room to express more for his next feed.

During moments of extreme despondency, I openly shared with family and friends how hard this separation from Isaac was. I just wanted to cuddle him at home, but there was no end date in sight. Some people hugged me or offered words of comfort. But many unwittingly dismissed me. They couldn't understand my pain. They reminded me that it was fortunate Isaac had survived. I didn't need reminding; I never will.

The highlight of each day in NICU was going into the warm laundry room with the premature babies' clothing and picking out a tiny bodysuit and sleepsuit for Isaac. The clothes were hung up on plastic hangers in order of size; some of them small enough for little dolls. This secret sanctuary provided a safe space to shed a tear in private with no one observing or judging me. I hated crying in front of people because I felt exposed. On down days, I intentionally sought out the potent, comforting fragrance of these freshly washed clothes. They felt smooth against my face, and the smell calmed my fatigued body. Closing my eyes and breathing deeply, I briefly shut out the world. These fleeting moments of solitude gave me the strength to face the busyness of the hospital, and our reality, once more.

Numerous friends and family members came to visit the hospital, welcoming Isaac into our lives and wishing us well. Much to their disappointment, they weren't allowed to touch him. Even a simple cold could have set Isaac's recovery back weeks, or worse. Of course, Giles and I wanted to see people; however, we were emotionally fragile and, after a while, their visits became too much. Not only did they interrupt our only time together each evening as a family, our one hour, but there were days when I wasn't coping. Days when I craved alone time with my newborn son, without having to meet the needs of other people. It was awkward to articulate this, and sometimes I didn't even want to. Other than Giles, nobody else understood the ache I felt in my heart whenever I left the hospital without Isaac. We made the unpopular decision to be honest and tell people we needed a break from visitors. Some understood and others didn't; I had to learn to live with their displeasure. It felt liberating to speak up for my own needs, and was a lesson in something I usually found difficult to do.

We sought solace from other parents, wanting to comprehend their situation and how they remained upbeat. Each account was similar, but at the same time entirely different.

"Visiting NICU has become a way of life for me," a mother explained to me at lunch one day. "I live over an hour from here and my other twin boy is already at home."

"How long has your son been in NICU?" I asked.

"One year," she replied.

When I heard this, my mouth dropped open. I felt humbled.

"Do you know when your son can go home?"

"No, he has a long road to recovery ahead of him. We're not sure when or if he will come home."

"I'm so sorry," I replied. "That must be devastating, I hope you are all reunited soon."

Hearing this news saddened me. While our situation was far from ideal, in comparison we were blessed, and it gave me the perspective I needed.

Some of the most traumatic memories I have of our time in NICU remain with me over sixteen years later. One day I heard quickened footsteps behind me and a voice shouting out: "Move please, coming through." Two male, pediatric doctors forced their way past me, running at full speed down the corridor as if their lives depended on it. In those moments they became superhuman, pushing a defenseless baby in an incubator to the safety of intensive care. Every second counted.

Observing my own and other's grief was a confronting part of life in NICU. Parents regularly cried and hugged next to their baby's incubator; it was a place where the best and worst news was received. I was not prepared for this. How could I be? The joy of hearing the words "Your baby can go home today" sharply contrasted with the devastation of hearing a baby had deteriorated. Silently watching parents crumble in front of me never got easier, no matter how many times I witnessed this. Not every baby survived. As hard as those moments were, I hope I never forget them because they remind me of how precious life is. We were the lucky ones; our story could have ended so differently. For this, I will be forever grateful.

CHAPTER 6

Isaac's First Wireless Cuddle

Breast is best, except when it's not.

Isaac started to improve, and he no longer needed his oxygen mask. Being moved out of intensive care into the high dependency unit was a major milestone, providing reassurance that we were closer to taking our baby home.

My heart always thumped with delight at the prospect of reaching inside the incubator, scooping Isaac up and pulling him close against my chest, breathing in the subtle fragrance of freshly washed clothes.

"Isaac," I'd whisper.

And then his beautiful eyes would open and gaze into mine with such love and tenderness, as if to say, "There you are. I've been waiting for you."

One Saturday morning, when Isaac was a few weeks old, Giles and I turned up together at the hospital. Walking into the hospital room, I looked toward Isaac's usual spot, but couldn't see him.

"Where is he? He's not here," I said.

My chest thudded and my mind raced, trying to make sense of it. "Oh no, this isn't good." Panic set in as I imagined the worst. Expressing milk every few hours throughout the night meant I was surviving on little sleep, and now my mind was playing tricks on me. Deducing Isaac had deteriorated but they hadn't been able to call us yet, I was too alarmed to ask the nurse what was going on.

The nurse looked over at us and smiled. "It's okay. Your son has been moved into the special care room. He just needs to learn how to feed and put some weight on, then he'll be able to go home."

"Really?" I replied with a massive sigh. "That's wonderful. I had no idea he was doing so well."

With Isaac making progress, there was pressure from the doctors and nurses to breastfeed, a prerequisite placed on me before Isaac could leave the hospital. The feeding tube was removed from Isaac's mouth and replaced with one going up inside his nose, past the throat and down into his stomach. Isaac's ability to suck was no longer hindered.

The incubators in the special care room were jammed close together, with little space to sit next to your baby. Isaac had developed further and was now sleeping in a hot cot which managed his body temperature and enabled him to maintain good weight gain. This was an exciting step forward because it allowed us to become more involved with Isaac's care.

I didn't have the most favorable relationship with my body at this stage. I hadn't fallen in love with it yet, and I was extremely self-conscious. The mere thought of stripping off in front of a room full of men and women to breastfeed filled my body with anxiety. Expressing milk in front of other women had been testing. But successfully breastfeeding felt like a bigger feat, one I was unequipped for emotionally and physically. *What happens if I do it wrong? Will I be able to produce enough milk for Isaac? Why aren't there any screens for me to hide behind? Will it hurt? Are the midwives going to be patient?* None of these concerns were conducive to learning such a vital skill, or enjoying what was supposed to be an intimate, bonding experience.

Feeding a premature baby who tired quickly was not easy. Firstly, I hadn't received any practical support from the nurses or midwives on the right technique, and secondly, Isaac invariably fell asleep. So when the maternal health nurse contacted me and offered to come to the hospital the next day to help, I welcomed her visit. In the end, though, she had no fresh advice on feeding a premature baby, and just became another pair of eyes watching me flounder. She asked a small Chinese nurse to help me, and she agreed with enthusiasm.

"I love the little dollies," the nurse laughed heartily, as she placed Isaac's mouth next to my exposed nipple.

Isaac carried on sleeping, so she brushed his mouth against my nipple to stimulate him to open it. As Isaac smelled my milk, he opened his eyes and firmly clamped down, latching on for the first time.

"Ow," I yelped, a sharp pain shooting through my body. "Should it hurt that much?"

"Oh yes, that's when you know they're on properly!" she shrieked with amusement. "It makes your toes curl, doesn't it!"

Unimpressed, I wondered how something so natural could be such agony. Rather than offering empathy, the nurse deemed my plight hilarious. In some respects, I found her endearing as she conveyed how much she loved caring for the miniature babies. But her breastfeeding support was limited, and sadly compromised my already wavering self-esteem.

One by one, each baby and their excited parents left special care, only to be immediately replaced with a smaller, sicker baby. Witnessing an African family's baby girl being struck down by a nasty virus just as they were able to leave the hospital made me realize how rapidly things could change, and not for the better. I appreciated how vulnerable all the babies were in the hospital, regardless of the fantastic care they received, and that the safest place for them was at home.

I was desperate for Isaac to be discharged, but unable to breastfeed him every four hours because there were no beds for me to stay in overnight. Isaac relied on his feeding tube during my absence. Until Isaac could feed consistently without this tube, and put on weight, I could not take him home. We were stuck in a vicious circle. Three weeks after Isaac's birth, we hit a brick wall.

Every time I left the hospital without Isaac my heart ached. I longed to enjoy my first cuddle with him alone, away from the noise, and was determined to make this happen. One afternoon I overheard a conversation that rapidly changed our situation.

"Am I able to bottle-feed my daughter?" a mother timidly asked one of the nurses.

"Yes. We're not able to recommend bottle-feeding, even if you bottle-feed expressed milk, as this is against hospital policy. We can only encourage and support breastfeeding."

"Oh," the mother said sounding perplexed.

I nudged Giles, encouraging him to also listen to the conversation.

"But now you've asked us, we can discuss it. Your baby will go home much sooner if you bottle-feed. She'll be less tired from sucking so will be able to take more milk and put weight on faster."

Frustrated that there had been so much pressure to breastfeed and we hadn't been given this additional beneficial advice, Giles and I talked through both options. One, carry on as we were. Isaac would eventually learn to breastfeed, and a special bond would develop between us. He'd slowly put weight on and, when breastfeeding was established, Isaac would ultimately be able to leave. But, the longer he stayed in the hospital, the greater the risk of picking up an infection that could compromise his immune system and delay his development. Or two, continue expressing milk and give it to him in a bottle. Feeding like this would take me twice as long, but at least expressing was now tolerable. Putting on weight quicker would more than likely mean Isaac could go home sooner. In truth, did it matter how he received my breast milk?

Logically it seemed like an easy decision, but for six months the guilt of giving up on breastfeeding and the special bonding with Isaac was incessant. Every time I fed him, I felt as though people were judging me. There was part of me that wanted to explain myself to them. That it was breast milk, not formula. That my son had been born prematurely and I had done what was right for my new family. Now I realize that the couples in hospital and my antenatal group were preoccupied with their own newborn dramas, and probably weren't bothered what I was doing. But at the time, my self-criticism was harsh. I felt disappointment in myself and therefore presumed others must too.

When my milk supply couldn't keep up with Isaac's demands, and he was still hungry after each feed, I needed to top him up with formula. Yet again I felt like a failure. I wish I had sought support from other new mothers who weren't breastfeeding to gain the reassurance that as long as Isaac was satisfied and growing, it didn't matter which type of milk he received. Joining online communities outside the hospital environment would have helped me see that my insecurities were normal, but that I was being exceptionally hard on myself. Rather, I was doing the best I could for both Isaac and me under difficult circumstances.

So following my conversation with Giles that day about the best way to feed our son, I cautiously asked the same midwife whether I could start bottle-feeding Isaac. I was incredibly reluctant to ask the question, but this inquiry was the turning point in Isaac's development. He started to stay awake for longer, which helped him grow and get stronger. I kicked myself for not asking more questions sooner. I hadn't wanted to seem ungracious about the care my son was receiving. Shortly after this, the doctors advised us we could sleep at the hospital with Isaac, "room in" as it was called, for the next two nights. Isaac would not be attached to any monitors or machines, and we would be wholly responsible for his care. The thought of experiencing my first cuddle without being surrounded by a room full of people was wonderful. But the best news was that if he hadn't lost weight and was doing well, we could take him home in three days!

Rushing to our house to get all the things we would need for our overnight stay, I couldn't get back to the hospital soon enough. When the doctor gave us the nod, we wheeled Isaac out of the special care nursery in his cot, around the corner to one of the rooms where we would spend the next forty-eight hours. Now it was just the three of us. As we closed the door on the hustle and bustle of the hospital, it slowly occurred to me how dependent we had become on the nurses and their reassurances. So while it was exciting to be in that hospital room, it was scary too. We had spent no time alone with Isaac and all his needs had been met straight away. He had barely cried. Now the fun started as we began learning how to properly care for our baby boy.

With tears in my eyes, our first proper cuddle was inexplicable. I discovered what I had been missing out on for the past four weeks. Isaac seemed so content in my arms without all the wires, and his little body rose and fell against mine in perfect rhythm. His feeding continued to go well, and Isaac took his bottles of expressed milk throughout the evening and night without any fuss. It was satisfying to be the one to attend to his cries at 2:00 a.m.–the one feed we had always missed.

The following morning, we pushed Isaac's cot back into special care. He needed to be weighed and checked over to make sure all was okay. If he was, we could all go back into the hospital room for the next twenty-four hours. My heart leaped with joy. We were closer to taking Isaac home. I carefully undressed Isaac, praying he had not lost weight. As we sat and watched the doctor place him on the weighing scales and wait for the verdict, the doctor calmly said, "Isaac can go home now."

I thought I had imagined it. Giles and I both looked at each other with disbelief. "What, right now?"

"Yes." He laughed.

I nearly passed out.

Elated and unable to stop smiling, I wondered if I was dreaming. Because we hadn't expected this fantastic news so soon, we didn't even have the car seat. So we rushed back to our house to pack all Isaac's things, including his cute going-home outfit. We fitted the car seat and drove back to the hospital like we were attending an emergency!

When we returned, I undressed Isaac from his hospital clothes for the last time. I pulled out his white-and-fawn matching teddy bear top and pant outfit. It was so soft but still too big. Isaac had lots of growing to do.

Carefully placing him in his car seat while he continued to sleep, we said thank you and goodbye to all the doctors and nurses. Our joy was tinged with sadness as I looked at all the other parents still waiting, but we felt immense gratitude that our turn had finally come. On the 14th of February–Valentine's Day–2006, Isaac left the hospital, and that night enjoyed his first proper bath in our lounge in front of a warm, open fire.

CHAPTER 7

Life Moves On

*You never know where an opportunity will lead you;
be courageous and embrace the adventure.*

We settled into life as a new family, pleased that the worst part was now firmly behind us. Friends and family enjoyed their first proper cuddles and posed for photos with the smallest baby they had ever seen. Some days, sleep deprivation and the usual newborn dramas were a real test. Isaac's colic and reflux meant we were frequently on the receiving end of projectile vomit, and developmental delays were part and parcel of life with a premature baby. But despite these things, I was filled with gratitude that we got to take our son home.

When Isaac was two months old, Giles was presented with an unexpected but exciting offer for our family to move to Shanghai in China for six to twelve months. If Isaac had been born around his due date, we couldn't have considered it. Always a firm believer that everything happens for a reason, even when it's hard, I knew we should embrace this opportunity. It was no coincidence that the right circumstances had lined up for us to be able to pursue this secondment while I was on maternity leave.

In August 2006, when Isaac was eight months old, we left the UK and moved into our two-story townhouse in Shanghai. We were fully committed to immersing ourselves in a different culture and endeavored to create many positive memories. Weekends were spent investigating this fascinating city and witnessing how people genuinely lived. I loved wandering around the old town and laughed as the locals surreptitiously (or so they thought) took photos of me. Some brave souls cautiously approached me, gesturing for their picture to be captured with this strange-looking Western woman. Being only a size six and 163 centimeters tall, I had never previously felt self-conscious of my body size or experienced people commenting on what I looked like. This small insight was an important lesson into what so many women with PCOS put up with, and how quickly we judge another person's appearance.

I learned a lot of resilience during our six-month secondment; little did I know how much I would need this skill over the forthcoming years. Living in a crowded, noisy city, where boundaries and personal space were not respected, became exhausting. Isaac received non-stop attention because of his now-blond hair and blue eyes. Strangers would wake him up and take him out of his pram multiple times a day. I never got used to the fact that traffic ignored the flashing green man, and taxi drivers often dumped Isaac and me on the side of busy roads when they changed their mind mid-journey about taking us home. All these situations kept me on high alert.

The most serious issue was that Shanghai's pollution and frequent smog aggravated Isaac's chest and he suffered from numerous episodes of bronchiolitis. Chest problems were common for premature babies due to their undeveloped lungs, but one night it was so bad Isaac almost ended up being admitted to the hospital. Disconcertingly, he needed to receive regular, ongoing doses of steroids. He had also not learned to crawl and was behind developmentally with his coordination and balance, despite learning to walk around twelve months old. So when the six months ended and we were offered an extension to our contract, we prioritized Isaac's health and returned to the UK. A secondary factor was that we were actively trying to have another baby and didn't want to lose out on any future maternity benefits from my current employer. My dream was to have four children, all close together in age. Having recently had Isaac, I saw no reason why this wouldn't happen. But life had other ideas.

Reflecting upon the choices we made, our Shanghai secondment turned out to be a significant part of a much bigger plan that we couldn't decipher at the time.

As Steve Jobs said, "You can't connect the dots looking forward; you can only connect them looking backward. So you have to trust that the dots will somehow connect in your future." Shanghai provided a notable way to encounter the highs and lows of living overseas with minimal risk and became a dress rehearsal for the real thing some years later. Synchronicity also played out in the form of a friendship with a Norwegian family, and a subsequent holiday to Norway. This country later became center stage for our infertility battle, an unwelcome battle for which we were ill-equipped.

Although I initially felt confident that it was only a matter of time before we would be blessed with another child and sibling for Isaac, the months began to pass by. Pressure in my job continued to rise and it was problematic to strike a healthy work-life balance. I became desperate to resign so I could reduce stress which was detrimental to my well-being and ability to conceive. But financially this wasn't an option for us. I felt trapped in my job. Part-time HR roles were hard to find, particularly at my grade. If I left now, I would lose the generous company maternity benefits giving me paid time at home with my future baby. I just needed to fall pregnant and everything would be resolved!

Family, friends and work colleagues announced their pregnancies. Despite being happy for them, it became a constant reminder about what my own body was failing to do. My sadness was becoming harder to ignore. Increasing despondency started to impact day-to-day life. Logically I knew this was counterproductive. But at this point, I lacked the tools and knowledge to stop the cycle. My deep desire to have another baby became all I could think about. These thoughts played on a repetitive loop in my mind. I struggled to switch off and focus on other things.

When my sleep began to be disturbed, I realized it was time to address this. Determined to find an alternative approach to manage debilitating stress and improve my chances of falling pregnant naturally, I began to research relaxation techniques. Meditation is where I started. I had been curious about meditation for many years, partly due to claims that it could transform my mind and my life. This decision was a significant turning point. I enrolled in a meditation course at my local Buddhist center and, for the first time, I experienced a sense of peace within myself that I had never known existed. Meditating in nature heightened the feelings of calm, and my connection with the great outdoors began in earnest.

I encourage you to read more about this in Part Two. Here I share meditation techniques and tips, and the benefits of immersing yourself in nature to immediately bring more tranquility into your life.

CHAPTER 8

Miscarriage Misery

You didn't stay for long, but you left an imprint on my heart.

M editation and being in nature helped me to cope better with infertility and work difficulties. At first, it was easier to brush off my growing concerns that I hadn't fallen pregnant and keep things in perspective. But after eighteen months, I allowed doubt to creep in. As each month came and went, I felt increasingly guilty. Guilty that I couldn't give Isaac a brother or sister; he talked about it often. Guilty that I was failing as a wife. Even though Giles was nothing other than patient and compassionate, I knew how much he wanted another child. Giles was regularly working away from home which didn't help. I rarely had a period and didn't know where I was in my cycle. It became harder to remain upbeat about conceiving.

Toward the end of February, 2008, I reluctantly booked a doctor's appointment to talk through my infertility issues. This was a big decision for me. I was desperate to avoid drugs, which were the next course of action to help me conceive. I had always struggled to swallow tablets, and refused to take painkillers unless the pain was intense because my body was quite sensitive to medication. After hearing the options though, I felt I had little choice. I left the surgery with a prescription for Metformin, a drug used by women who suffer from PCOS to treat insulin dysfunction, regulate blood sugar, hormone irregularities, and ovulation. As with most drugs, there are side effects, and I didn't enjoy the daily upset stomach and nausea.

At this point, I was working at a university in Bristol as a HR adviser. My role was to support the deans and their academic staff with any people issues. One of the campuses was set in a serene sanctuary filled with trees and fields, a real perk of my job. Each visit I walked through the trees as this gave me time to get out of my head and be still before the busy day began. This ritual became a significant part of my meditation practice. During one of my early morning walks, through tears I prayed, asking to be blessed with another baby. At that moment I surrendered, and completely opened myself up to what my future held. In my heart, I knew that I was now ready to be a loving mom again. I felt sure the timing was right.

Coincidentally, as part of the university's well-being program that month, we were fortunate to be able to try a range of alternative therapy sessions during work hours. Given how keen I was to come off the drugs, and my positive reflexology sessions as a teenager, I didn't hesitate to book an appointment with a reflexologist. I needed some "me" time to help me unwind and manage my PCOS better.

At lunchtime, I walked over to the university campus and located the small meeting room where my session was taking place. It lacked natural light but was quiet and cozy enough. The therapist had set up in the corner of the room, next to the table and four chairs that filled the rest of the area. He had a beard and kind eyes, and I immediately warmed to him.

While the therapist worked on my feet, we chatted about the reasons why I had booked an appointment.

"I need help to de-stress and unwind," I explained.

"Yes, life can be hectic," he empathetically replied.

"I'm also wanting to have another baby, but it isn't happening for us."

As the treatment progressed the therapist paused briefly. Something had caught his attention.

"Your uterus is hot," he said with surprise. "I don't know what that means. It hasn't come up in a session before."

Assuming the heat must be due to my significant hormone imbalances or the Metformin I'd been taking, I put our conversation aside. Returning to work,

I felt brighter and more relaxed, which was just what I needed. But when I got home, I pondered whether I could be pregnant (as unlikely as this was). I was nauseous, but then again this could just be the medication. After much internal debate, I decided that ruling pregnancy out would enable me to refocus on getting myself in a prime position to fall pregnant. I walked upstairs to the bathroom and undid the wrapper on one of the numerous cheap pregnancy tests I had brought back from Shanghai. After using the test, I carefully placed it down on the side of the bath and washed my hands. I had been here so many times before and the potential disappointment was much to bear; I resigned myself to another negative result. But to my utter disbelief, a second line slowly appeared on the pregnancy test. *How could this be?* After eighteen months, at long last, I was pregnant again. Physically shaking with excitement and relief, I ran downstairs to show the result to Giles. My prayers had been answered, and I was ecstatic.

On cloud nine, all my previous failures and troubles disappeared, and I started planning all things baby-related, including re-establishing Isaac's bedroom as a nursery. At my doctor's appointment, I was advised to stop taking Metformin, ironically having already been pregnant when I started taking it the previous week. I got a referral for a dating scan to confirm how many weeks pregnant I was. This was an opportunity for us to see our tiny baby's heartbeat for the first time. I couldn't wait.

The day of the hospital appointment arrived. Giles helped me to lie on the couch and gel was put on my stomach. It was chilly, but I didn't mind. The sonographer worked in silence while we waited with anticipation to see our baby's heartbeat appear on the screen. The silence continued for what felt like an eternity. *What's going on? This is taking a long time. Stop being impatient. For goodness sake Sarah, relax.*

Finally, the stinging words, "I'm so sorry–there's no heartbeat," abruptly ended the silence, and the pregnancy.

"What do you mean?" I had to say it, even though I knew exactly what she meant.

"It looks like your baby stopped growing a few weeks ago," she explained. "I'm sorry."

Everything slowed right down, I was taken aback to hear that my baby had already died. Utter devastation swept through my body, and a small piece of my spirit felt as though it had floated away like smoke from a campfire on a windy day. My heart ached, and shattering waves of shock and sadness rushed through my body. Too ashamed to look at Giles, I turned my head, tears filling my eyes. I knew how excited Giles had been about the prospect of becoming a father again, and now my damaged body had put an end to this. *This can't be. She's made a mistake. It's not supposed to be like this.*

After about five minutes the sonographer left the room to speak to the support nurse. I wiped the gel off my stomach with trembling hands and got dressed. I began to assimilate the news. *What did I do wrong? How has this happened?* I wondered whether this was because I had stopped taking Metformin, a drug that I would find out years later can lower the risk of miscarriage. It seemed coincidental that everything was fine and then a week later it was all over. I knew these questions were a waste of time, but it didn't stop the desire for answers.

The support nurse returned and explained we would move to a different room to talk. I felt like a failure. We followed her into a long corridor filled with expectant mothers waiting to hear their fate. Some of them looked doubtful and anxious; perhaps they had been here before. Others seemed jovial, clearly as unprepared for any potential bad news as I had been. I turned my gaze away from them, envious that they were pregnant and I wasn't. The nurse quietly ushered us into a cold, uninviting room and we sat down, still dazed. For privacy, the blue curtain was drawn across the rectangular window in the door. The nurse handed me a box of tissues and sat down opposite us.

"How are you?" she asked me softly.

"Not good, to be honest," I replied despondently. "It has taken us so long to get to this point, and now we're right back at the beginning. I don't understand what happened."

She looked at Giles who sat next to me holding my hand. "Sad," was the only word that came out of his mouth.

I noticed that the nurse's face was round and warm, with small glasses snug across her nose. I instantly liked her, and she seemed genuinely sorry that we were having this conversation.

"There's nothing you could have done differently," she said. "You've had a 'missed miscarriage'. Do you know what that is?"

I shook my head as she began to explain the difference between this and a normal miscarriage.

Miscarriage is a term many people are familiar with. According to the Royal Women's Hospital in Victoria, Australia, a miscarriage occurs when a pregnancy stops growing. Eventually, the pregnancy tissue will pass out of the body.[2]

A missed miscarriage, however, also called a "silent miscarriage" or "missed abortion," is a type of pregnancy loss (before twenty weeks) that can be hard to detect without an ultrasound scan. The pregnancy has stopped growing but the tissue has not passed and there is still a sac (the structure surrounding the embryo or fetus) in the uterus.[3] Even though there is no heartbeat and the fetus has died, the body does not recognize the pregnancy loss or expel the pregnancy tissue. As a result, the placenta may keep releasing hormones so the woman could continue to experience signs of pregnancy.[4]

The nurse carried on talking while my mind repeatedly wandered off. I felt like I was silently observing a scene of someone else's life playing on a large screen.

"It's impossible to know when your body will have a miscarriage," the nurse explained. "In the meantime, the sac still grows, and you may feel pregnant because of the pregnancy hormones."

"Oh great," I laughed sarcastically, deflecting my sadness.

"You need to be aware that the pregnancy could go on for weeks. When you do have a miscarriage, you may have cramps and vaginal bleeding. Passing the tissue could be very painful and upsetting; you may be able to identify parts of your baby. I'm sorry to be so graphic, but I need to be honest with you. There is also a risk that the miscarriage will not entirely complete, and you will need to come into the hospital for minor surgery to have the remaining tissue removed."

"Okay, I understand," I replied sobbing. There was nothing else to say.

Despite the nurse being incredibly supportive, her words brought me little comfort, and I wanted to reject the numbness that was taking over my body. It was helpful to get my head around what was happening and why, but it was hell still feeling pregnant, knowing that my baby had already died. The reality set in that we had waited more than eighteen months for this pregnancy, and now my body had failed not just me, but all three of us.

"You have two options, Sarah. You can wait for a miscarriage and the pregnancy tissue to be expelled naturally, which is important to some women, or I can book you in next week for a Dilation and Curettage (D&C). I will leave you alone to discuss this between yourselves and come back in five minutes." The nurse left the room.

D&C, as it is commonly known, is a minor operation that is done in an operating room, usually under general anesthetic. There is no cutting involved because the surgery happens through the vagina. The cervix (neck of the womb) is gently opened and the remaining pregnancy tissue is removed so that the uterus is empty.[5]

The decision rested with me as it was my body, but I appreciated having Giles there to support me. I was aware that any surgical procedure, no matter how routine, came with a small risk. I had never been under general anesthetic before, so I wasn't sure how my body would react or what to expect afterwards. However, in my heart, I knew that for my healing and mental sanity I needed to opt for surgery.

"What have you decided?" the nurse enquired when she returned.

"I want to get this over and done with, so I'll come into hospital."

"I've got good news," she said. "There's a hospital bed available next week."

It didn't feel like good news. With mixed emotions, we booked the appointment and left the hospital. I was in pieces.

I had already taken a few hours off work so I needed to go straight to the office to explain my absence to my boss. It was a heavy conversation and one I would have preferred not to have, mainly as I hadn't been in my job long. I was concerned that it would affect my career to reveal plans for another baby. Thankfully though, my manager was supportive, gave me time off work, and remains a friend over fourteen years later.

The mere thought of being in a hospital filled me with dread, let alone the reason for the hospital admittance. Still nauseous, sore and tired, I was emotionally crippled but unable to articulate this, even to Giles. The day before my appointment for the D&C, I returned to the hospital to have a repeat ultrasound to double-check whether the sonographer had got it wrong. To my despair, there was still no heartbeat–the procedure would go ahead as planned the next day.

The following morning, hungry and filled with anxiety, I looked around the crowded hospital waiting room. There were girls sat with their mothers, and others with their friends. One by one, they left the waiting area. After about fifteen minutes, my name was called. Entering the ward, the same girls occupied the beds around mine. They were chattering loudly and smiling. I could not join in.

An oversized hospital gown was handed to me to put on, and I placed my clothes on the chair next to my bed. After about an hour, the doctors came around to talk to us all about our surgery. Regardless of the muffled conversations, it became obvious the girls were undergoing abortions. This was effectively the same procedure as mine, just carried out for other reasons. Again, the loss hit me. It was as if the wrong baby had been put inside the wrong body. I didn't judge these girls–I understood they were at different stages of their lives–but salt was being rubbed into an open wound.

As I reluctantly signed the consent form, knowing there was no going back, no miracle to be had, I was advised that the remains of my pregnancy would be kept by the hospital. There was part of me that wanted to see them, so this whole situation would seem less dreamlike. But part of me also knew that those visions would have stayed with me, and probably not helped my grief.

I lay on the hospital bed in the fetal position as the hours ticked by. Giles and I didn't speak. There was nothing more to say. Every ounce of my being wanted to be anywhere else apart from there. Knowing it would soon be over was a mixture of relief and further grief. All hope lost. I would be left to pick up the pieces once more. The thought of being completely unaware of what was happening to me while lying on an operating table made me vulnerable. I was concerned about how well my body would tolerate a general anesthetic. How would I be when I woke up, and, worse still, whether I'd wake up at all. This fear was illogical but deep-rooted.

After some time, the hospital staff came to collect me, pushing me in my bed down the corridor to the operating room. The matter-of-fact anesthetist asked my name and date of birth, but he was reassuring nonetheless. Hospital staff stood on both sides of the bed as the general anesthetic slowly pumped through my body, and I counted backward from ten to one. My last memory was staring intently at the array of bright lights on the ceiling.

When I slowly awoke from my D&C procedure, I became aware I had no underwear on. I felt exposed and violated, as though I had been tampered with. There was a sizable sanitary towel pushed between the top of my bare legs, and the hospital gown felt cold and uncomfortable against my skin. I had no memory of what had just occurred; I couldn't wait to get dressed and leave the hospital.

Relief at the operation being over didn't last long as I remembered that my pregnancy had ended, and we were right back at the beginning. Bleeding and wretched, my one small glimmer of hope was the reassurance that this procedure would force my body into a regular cycle for at least the next month. Perhaps we'd get a vague idea of when I could be ovulating, which was something.

"How are you, Sarah?" one of the nurses asked.

I started to cry.

"Would you like to speak to the hospital chaplain?" she said. "It may help you."

As a spiritualist, even as a young child, I have believed in an energy, a higher force, that connects us all. So I was guided to say, "Yes, please." Despite being aware it would delay my departure from the hospital, it felt right to accept her offer. With nothing to lose except time, I was sure this conversation would help me to process my grief faster.

An hour later the chaplain came to see me. She sat on the chair next to my bed, and Giles left us to converse in private.

"Hello Sarah, how are you?"

"Devastated," I replied without hesitation.

"I'm sorry for the loss of your baby. It's a difficult time," the chaplain responded.

I was surprised that the chaplain had referred to my miscarriage as a baby. I did feel as though I had lost a baby, a future child, even though he or she had been so tiny and hadn't properly formed. The chaplain was the first person to acknowledge my loss, and one of the only people who ever genuinely did. I was blessed to have her support. Maybe she had been through this herself, but regardless of the reasons why, it was just what I needed to hear as I tried to make sense of it all.

"I'm failing to understand what the point to all this is. What's the bigger purpose? Will I ever know?"

"Yes, one day you'll understand why this has happened. Until then, keep trusting. It doesn't feel like it right now, but there is hope," the chaplain consoled me. "Would you like to write in the chapel's book of condolences?"

Grateful for "Baby Willoughby" to be acknowledged, writing in the book was one of my saddest moments; it all seemed so final. My words on the page stared back at me with such emptiness, marking the end of another chapter.

Baby Willoughby

7ᵗʰ March, 2008

So small, so special, we will always remember you. Always in our thoughts and hearts, we know you would have become an amazing person.

We will meet one day, until then, all our love.

Mommy and Daddy.

The chaplain's compassion validated my emotions and permitted me to grieve. As she listened, she didn't judge or try to offer a solution; she was just there with me in that moment, holding space for me to feel whatever I felt. Today I am still thankful for our conversation.

Driving home was painful; I hadn't expected to be so sore from such minor surgery. Emotionally dazed, there were no words to explain how much I wished this was not real. As we turned into our street and I slowly walked up the steep stone steps to my house, lying outside my front door was a small, pretty bunch of flowers and a card from my friend Delphine. This meant so much to me. It warmed my heart that someone cared.

Upon entering the house, I needed to be alone and went upstairs for a rest, curling up on my bed in the fetal position for the second time that day, devastated. I knew tears would help, but no tears came. I was met only by complete emptiness.

Why am I so flawed? What have I done wrong? Yet in my heart, I knew I would get through this somehow. I had to, for the sake of my son. Right now, I couldn't imagine when or how. I figured this tear-jerking torment wouldn't stop anytime soon. We had come so close, but my baby had slipped through my fingers.

My husband came upstairs to talk.

"Hi, how are you?"

"Sad," I replied. "Numb."

"I'm sorry," he said. "I wish there was something I could do to change things."

"I'm not sure how I'll get through this," I whispered with tears rolling down my cheeks. "I hate feeling like this." I looked toward Giles. "How are you?"

"I'm sad. But we need to try to put this behind us and focus on the future. It's for the best," Giles replied as he stood looking out of the bedroom window.

I knew he was right, but a switch flicked in my mind. I was angry and disillusioned. Regardless of Giles's underlying sadness, he had already mentally moved on. Envious of this, I longed to be in that place with him, to escape the intense emotions that I was feeling. I logically understood we all deal with things differently, and it was normal for Giles to be less attached to the pregnancy. He had not dealt with the pregnancy hormones. He hadn't felt the physical changes or the life of our future child growing inside him. However, I hadn't expected this moving on to happen so soon, and my envy turned to resentment. I had hoped we could support each other through our pain; this is not how I had envisaged it would be. Today I'm able to look at this situation with fresh eyes.

"Please leave," I sobbed.

"Why?" Giles asked.

"I just need to be alone. You don't get it."

Confused, he walked out of the room, closed the door behind him and I cried myself to sleep.

A few days later the chaplain phoned me to ask how I was doing. It was reassuring someone cared enough to make that call. I was still distraught, especially when talking about it, but the conversation offered something entirely out of the blue.

"I wondered if you would like me to organize a private funeral service and cremation for your baby?"

In biological terms, our baby was not even a baby, so I was quite taken aback and honored by such a kind-hearted gesture. I couldn't believe that someone, anyone, wanted to acknowledge my child's life and pay tribute to what could have been.

When I had collected my thoughts I replied, "Yes, that would be lovely, thank you. When were you thinking?"

"Friday the 14th of March. I will be in touch tomorrow to confirm the details."

I smiled to myself as I remembered that the 14th of March had been Isaac's due date. Now this date would be even more meaningful.

Turning up at the Chapel of Rest the following week, my stomach churned.

"Hello Sarah, Giles. You must be Isaac." The chaplain welcomed us into the chapel. Isaac was only two years old and too young to grasp the significance of the occasion. The chaplain handed me a simple white service sheet with "Funeral Service for Baby Willoughby" typed on the front in blue above a photo of a yellow daffodil. With leaden hearts, we sat down on the firm, wooden pews at the front, the chapel suddenly feeling enormous and quiet.

The chaplain approached Giles and asked, "Would you like to carry the coffin?"

Giles was initially stunned but agreed at once. He walked to the back of the chapel, and was handed the smallest wooden coffin I have ever seen. The coffin was less than a foot long. As I watched Giles walk down the aisle toward me, the coffin looked even smaller in his hands. It was flawless. The words, "Baby Willoughby" were engraved on a gold plaque on top.

Music played softly in the background. Desperately trying to fight back the tears, I looked away in case I completely broke down. I didn't want Isaac to see me upset; he needed to be shielded from my desolation.

The words, poems and songs shared in the remembrance service filled me with such sorrow and deep gratitude. I share some of these here in the hope that they provide comfort to you or others.

Introduction

We have come here to honor with dignity a little one whose birth you had been anticipating for just a short time, and perhaps we come to share in some way our feelings of loss of this child. We gather here with a real hope that through this time together, we can remember your baby without fear or guilt or desperation and then hand your little one on to God with gentle care and confidence.

Opening Prayer

Eternal God, whose love knows no end, please help us through this service to know that you are close to us. As we hear your words, may our hearts and minds feel comforted by the assurance that Baby Willoughby is safe in your care.
We ask this through Jesus Christ our Lord. Amen.

Our Thoughts and Prayers

We support you, Sarah and Giles
with our love and prayers.
Faced with all the emotions that the loss
of your little one has brought,
we pray that you may be given courage and
help in your pain and grief.
We think of all families who live with
the loss of a child before their due time.
May they be comforted and find a way
to peace in their minds and hearts.

Commendation

Little one
into the freedom of the wind and sunshine
we let you go.
Into the dance of the stars and planets
we let you go.
Into the wind's breath and the hands of the creator
we let you go.
We want you to be happy, to be free,
go safely, go dancing, go running home.

These words reinforced that our baby's life was meaningful. It also gave me that much-needed chance to say goodbye. As the service came to an end and the coffin started to move away, the curtain slowly closed. I watched it disappear with the remains of my baby inside, and I broke down in tears. I cried for what could have been, and for the child I would not meet. My heart had been ripped in two.

CHAPTER 9

Hospital Drama
(I Wish This Was Just a TV Show)

Nothing can prepare you for your own mortality.

The grief and trauma I experienced in my private life both coincided with, and amplified, the dissatisfaction I felt in my professional life. My infertility and personal issues became the catalyst for beginning to open my eyes to the glaringly obvious. Deep down, I knew I needed to leave my job, but I was still too scared to take this leap of faith. I was also completely distracted by my desire to have another baby. Meditation continued to open my heart and I began soul-searching, interrogating the meaning of life, my life. As I started to do this my views about myself, my aspirations and the world in general slowly began to shift, though I still had no idea where it was taking me. At the right time, it would all be revealed. In the meantime, I needed to be patient.

Months went by and I began losing hope. Following my miscarriage, I had been prescribed Metformin again to regulate my menstrual cycle, and a new medication, Clomiphene. Clomiphene induces ovulation, egg production, in the ovaries. These drugs were not working though, and no more options were available without seeing a specialist, something I had been resisting. Not only did I not want to admit defeat, but I also had concerns that hospital treatment would increase the stress, frustration and pressure I already felt. Many months passed before I mustered up the courage to face the situation and visited my doctor for a hospital referral. After a brief chat, she handed me a letter for the fertility department, advising me it would be a six-month wait for the first appointment. Long waiting lists were the reality of receiving treatment under the NHS.

In August 2008, my husband and I arrived at the hospital and were told to wait in the gynecology department waiting room. The registrar eventually called my name.

"Before we start," I said, "I just want to ask why I'm being seen in the gynecology department? My referral was for the fertility department."

"Because we need to try some of the drugs again and regulate your cycle," the registrar replied with disinterest. "We can do that in this department."

"I'm so confused. I've already tried every drug possible. We've been trying for a baby for years, and now you're telling me we need to go right back to the beginning and repeat everything." Clearly, I was exasperated. "We don't even know if I ovulate. Surely we should be checking that?"

"Please excuse me, I will be back in a moment," the registrar announced.

"Where's he going?" I asked Giles.

"I have no idea." Giles shrugged.

"We're not getting answers," I replied with frustration in my voice.

The registrar returned to the room and sat down. "I've just spoken to the gynecology and obstetrics consultant. I'm going to write you a prescription for Provera to regulate your menstrual cycle. Take it every forty days if you have a negative pregnancy test. We'll do some blood tests to establish if you're ovulating."

"Did you ask him whether I should be seen in this department or fertility?"

"No, I'm happy to see you here," the registrar replied, annoyed with my questions. "I will see you again in four months. In the meantime, you should try to fall pregnant naturally."

I felt as though something wasn't right, but I was getting nowhere. Giving up, I took the prescription from the registrar's hand, agreeing to return at the end of the year.

The registrar had instructed me to continue taking Metformin and Clomiphene. On day two to five of each menstrual cycle, I needed to book a blood test at the doctor's surgery to check my luteinizing hormone (LH) and follicle-stimulating hormone (FSH) levels, and again on day twenty-one to test progesterone levels. I knew taking time off work every month to do this would mean making my hours up at weekends, but I had no choice.

As each blood test for ovulation came back negative, gradually disillusion set in. We were getting nowhere. Bitterness built toward the drugs, medical appointments and potential future fertility treatment, and I knew there had to be a better way to manage this exasperating situation. I had heard that learning mindfulness-based approaches, and how to be fully present in each moment, could help me "live well with pain and stress."[6] In turn, I hoped my decision-making would be more positive and informed. In September 2008, I enrolled in a Breathworks mindfulness course held at the Buddhist center, where I'd previously attended weekly meditation classes. In Part Two of this book, I share how life-changing this practice turned out to be. It could be for you too.

In the months following the hospital appointment, I experienced yet further disappointment, and, more worryingly, mix-ups. In December, 2008, in my second appointment with the registrar, my concerns were not being heard–I was fobbed off. In hindsight, I should have asked more questions and stood my ground. Again, I asked why I wasn't attending the fertility department when I was actively trying to conceive. I suggested more tests to check my hormone levels to decipher what was happening to my body. The registrar begrudgingly left the room to speak to the consultant. Surprisingly, when he returned, I was instructed to see the nurse at the end of the corridor to carry out the requested blood tests.

The young nurse directed me to sit in the big, leather chair as she meticulously gathered all the needles and tubes, ready to draw my blood. I appreciated her gentle manner–it had been a long day. She strived to find a vein but each one silently caved in. I'd been poked, prodded and my entire arm was bruised. The hospital appointments had run late, and it was now almost 5:00 p.m. Having not eaten or drunk for many hours, my blood pressure was low. The room started spinning like a wheel. Wanting to vomit, I was overcome with an inordinate bout of pins and needles throughout my whole body. I couldn't communicate, lost total awareness of my body, and started to shake. This had never happened in all my years of blood tests. I was not in control, and it was like I was having an out-of-body experience.

"Are you okay, Sarah?" the nurse placed her hand on my arm.

Unable to speak, I remained silent.

"Sarah, can you hear me? Are you okay?"

Concerned for my welfare, the nurse went to the consultant's office, while Giles kept an eye on me. She returned with a glass of water and a biscuit. Apparently, I would be fine. Dehydration and the vein poking had got the better of me. I felt quite embarrassed. I didn't like being the center of attention in any situation.

To my surprise, five minutes later the consultant appeared in the room. He looked at my medical file and previous blood-test results, then scanned my pelvis for the first time, an ultrasound that should have been carried out years earlier. Within minutes he understood precisely what my issues were, and what help we needed next.

"Your ovaries are both enlarged, with multiple immature follicles on each," he said.

"Oh." This was not what I wanted to hear.

"Your ovaries have a very marked polycystic morphology."

Unsure what this meant, but certain it wasn't good news, I nodded quietly as he continued. "Your hormone levels are also extremely disturbed."

"I'm sorry Sarah, but the registrar isn't an expert on PCOS and has made some mistakes with your care. Although it has been appropriate for you to take Provera to induce a withdrawal bleed, with the appearance of your ovaries, you shouldn't have been taking this until fifty-six days after your cycle, and only if a pregnancy test was negative."

I sat up in bed and looked him directly in the eye. "What could have happened?"

"If you'd managed to fall pregnant while taking all the prescribed tablets, you could have accidentally induced a miscarriage."

I looked at him, outraged. This oversight was devastating. The consultant apologized for the substantial errors, admitting that my treatment had been unsatisfactory, and detrimental to both my physical and emotional well-being.

He confirmed that my appointments should have been in the fertility department where these errors would not have occurred.

"So, what happens now?" I asked, trying to find something positive among the doom and gloom.

"Based on what I've seen today and read in your notes, it's highly unlikely that you'll fall pregnant naturally. Even if you did, the probability of you maintaining the pregnancy would be slim."

I'd been right all along. But it didn't please me that this was the case. Intrauterine insemination (IUI) was not an option for us. This simple, less invasive form of fertility treatment helps the sperm inseminate the uterus close to the time of ovulation. However, due to my very disturbed hormone levels and age (being well under forty at the time), we were advised that the intricacies of controlling the cycle, and increased risk of ovary overstimulation, meant it was not safe to try.

"So that leaves you with two options. IVF or ovarian drilling," the consultant recommended. "As you've already conceived a child naturally, you won't qualify for one free round of IVF treatment. Ovarian drilling can be carried out free under the NHS but there's a waiting list of six to twelve months for this procedure."

IVF is a process of removing mature eggs from the woman's ovaries and fertilizing them with sperm in a test tube (in vitro). The fertilized egg undergoes embryo culture for two to six days and is then implanted in the uterus to establish a successful pregnancy. It takes roughly two weeks to complete one IVF cycle. Ovarian drilling is a surgical procedure done during laparoscopy under general anesthetic. An electrosurgical needle, or laser, is used to puncture the ovary four to ten times and destroy parts of the ovaries. This technique can trigger ovulation for six to twelve months and dramatically reduce male hormones in women who have PCOS. To be honest, I didn't fancy either of these options.

"So, what we need to do now is refer you to the fertility department. There is currently a four-month wait. We can then discuss your treatment with you further and carry out more tests." He tried to reassure me, but it didn't work.

"Can't you see me sooner, especially given all the mistakes?"

"Sorry, no."

"That's exceptionally disheartening," I replied, "Particularly under the circumstances."

Grabbing my coat, I left the hospital deflated and angry. *Was I fighting a losing battle? Perhaps a big family was not meant to be?* I wondered if I should give all my attention to Isaac, and put the idea of having another baby out of my mind altogether.

Returning home, I promised to refocus my despair into preparing myself for the next hospital appointment in 2009. But although I tried, I couldn't shift my concern that we were losing valuable time. And time wasn't on our side. Fright swooped in like a bird of prey catching its next victim. If we opted for the free ovarian drilling procedure, I would have to wait six to twelve months for the surgery, and it would only provide us with a small six-month window to conceive naturally. The other option was to take on the huge medical bills for IVF treatment. The pit of my stomach filled with tension as the expenses mounted up in my mind's eye. I had an inkling there must be another option, one we hadn't considered.

Some days later, once we had researched both options further, I began to investigate IVF in different clinics both within the UK and overseas. I'd lost all confidence in the local hospital and wasn't sure I was willing to risk receiving further inadequate medical treatment.

Once we started researching which hospitals and clinics were available in the UK for IVF treatment, we discovered it was expensive. We could afford one IVF cycle, but if the procedure was unsuccessful, saving up the money for another round was going to prove tricky. This made us feel slightly defeated before we'd even begun. Not willing to give up, we decided to research alternatives. I joined online forums and read reviews for IVF centers. To my surprise, the same IVF clinic in Norway kept coming up positively. I decided to investigate further.

Having recently returned from a holiday in Norway, we had excellent insight into the country and culture, and had warmed to the Norwegian people. We also admired their professionalism and excellent health care. If an opportunity ever arose, we'd even agreed that we would pursue a secondment there.

Further exploration highlighted that the clinic had short waiting lists, excellent facilities, high success rates and affordable prices, even taking the additional costs of flights and accommodation into account. This meant that I could be pregnant before we had even attended our first IVF appointment in Bristol. In

Norway, the team of fertility specialists and nurses was small, so I'd see the same people throughout the whole cycle. Given the stress involved in IVF, the prospect of being treated less like a number was distinctly appealing.

In January 2009, after further discussion, we booked an initial short trip to visit the clinic and meet the IVF team. Following more ultrasound scans, we discerned this was our best possibility to have another baby. Regardless of all the reassurance we received, we knew it was not going to be easy. The likelihood of success was low. I wasn't keen on injecting myself with fertility drugs and was concerned about the potential side effects of doing so, but it seemed like a small price to pay for the chance of having another baby and sibling for Isaac.

Impressed by both the clinic and the medical professionals, we agreed in principle to start IVF. I was given all the information about where to purchase the fertility drugs in the UK, and began taking the pill to regulate my cycle. As we prepared for our return to Norway in March, we decided to turn the trip into a family holiday and have something fun to look forward to once the whole IVF process was completed. It also ensured I would be less tense, giving the embryos the best chance to implant. Returning to work too soon could have compromised our chances of seeing a positive pregnancy test after the torturous two-week wait. My mother-in-law kindly agreed to accompany us to Norway, to look after Isaac when we were at the clinic and provide us with some support. At the time we had no idea how major this decision would be.

IVF turned out to be a tumultuous emotional rollercoaster. My hormones were haywire, the various drugs unpleasant, and the needles tremendously painful. Giles reluctantly administered the injections into my stomach. He repeatedly apologized for hurting me, knowing how much it stung, even though it was for a good cause. I was not good at deliberately inflicting pain on myself so there was no choice!

Throughout the IVF cycle, I swung from hope to excitement to worry to fear. Good days were followed by many more bad days. Self-criticism crept in as I perceived my body had failed to do one of the most natural things in life: conceive a baby. The scariest part of IVF was allowing myself to be cautiously excited that within six weeks I might be pregnant. The flipside would be dealing with another failure and being back at the drawing board again.

Before I started taking the fertility drugs, I knew I needed to support myself through the IVF treatment so we had a higher chance of success. I followed my intuition and booked myself some hypnotherapy sessions at a local clinic with a lady called Maddie. A year or so before, a leaflet had come through the door with her details. Now I knew why I had kept it.

I loved the name Maddie. We would have called our first child Maddie if Isaac had been a girl. I knew hypnotherapy could help me cope with the highs and lows of IVF, and keep me reasonably rational. I believed that how you think affects how you feel. Meditation had already profoundly changed my life for the better, and I was sure hypnotherapy could do the same. I expected some discomfort during the egg collection. Unlike in the UK, it was done under a local anesthetic, not a general. I needed to be relaxed and upbeat during this procedure and the embryo transfer.

The many stages of the IVF cycle went well, but as I came closer to finishing injecting the fertility drugs into my stomach, I became aware of some discomfort in my abdomen. It wasn't acute, but I had this niggling doubt that something was wrong. Emailing the clinic put my mind at rest as they didn't seem too bothered. I finished the course of drugs, packed our bags and flew to Norway with the family.

In IVF, the ovaries are stimulated so that the follicles grow and produce mature eggs. An ultrasound then determines which is the right day to undertake the egg collection. On average, a woman typically produces around ten to twelve follicles during an IVF cycle (depending on age, medical history and response to stimulation).

As I lay on the couch in the hospital for an ultrasound to check how many follicles had developed, I heard the fertility specialist quietly mutter "Oh dear" under his breath.

"Is there a problem?" I asked.

"Your ovaries have reacted to the fertility drugs. They're overstimulated and are swollen which explains why you've been experiencing discomfort."

I tried to remain calm as the follicles were counted. The specialist confirmed that thirty had formed, which was many more than normal. I knew this wasn't a good thing, but he didn't seem too concerned. Despite the risk that after the follicles had been extracted the overstimulation could escalate and the egg transfer may not be possible, the egg collection was scheduled for a few days later.

After breakfast, I used my pill cutter to split the large painkillers into smaller pieces, so they were easier to swallow, and headed to the clinic. I was led into a large waiting room and given a blue gown to wear over my underwear. It tied up at the back but did not provide complete coverage and I felt self-conscious walking around the clinic in front of the other patients and their partners.

In the room where the egg collection was taking place, I was asked to remove my underwear and lie in a reclining chair with my legs in stirrups. All dignity was lost as I exposed myself to the medical staff involved. The room was freezing. I put my earphones in and played my hypnotherapy track, trying to block out what was happening. As the needles filled with local anesthetic pricked the tender tissue inside my vagina, again and again, I was hopeful that the worst was over.

The retrieval of the eggs was painful, and the razor-sharp scratching sensation continued much longer than usual due to the abnormally large number that needed to be collected. Thankfully, the hypnotherapy exercise relaxed me somewhat, as my mind drifted off to other places and I focused on the soft, reassuring words. After forty minutes, the last egg was extracted. Breathing a massive sigh of relief, and my heart filled with hope, I prayed that the eggs would grow into good-quality embryos and some would survive for the transfer process days later.

After the egg collection, I rested and recovered on a blue reclining chair while we waited for an update. I went to the toilet and placed a sanitary pad in my underwear to deal with the blood loss caused by all the prodding and poking. The specialist appeared in due course with the results.

"The good news is that everything went well, and we managed to remove many follicles from your ovaries. We'll call you to let you know how they're doing, their quality and grading," he said. "How's the discomfort today?"

"It's bearable."

"I need to tell you that because you're already overstimulating, the embryo transfer may not be able to go ahead later this week. I'm sorry," he replied.

My heart sank. "Really?"

"If implantation is successful and you become pregnant, managing the overstimulation becomes much more complicated because of the increased hormone levels. In extreme circumstances, it can seriously compromise your health and lead to a viable pregnancy needing to be terminated. If overstimulation continues, we'll freeze the embryos and you can return for implantation after you've recovered," the consultant advised.

Not wanting to cry in front of the other couples in the room, I pushed my tears aside. I knew there was not much chance of the embryo transfer taking place this visit. Even though I understood the reasons why, and agreed it would be the most sensible thing to do, I felt sad and despondent that things hadn't gone according to plan. Not only did it mean that the embryos would have to be frozen, which significantly reduced pregnancy-success rates, we'd also need to take more time off work to return to Norway later in the year. The extra costs for travel, accommodation and embryo storage also entered my thoughts.

"The most important thing is that you rest and allow your body to recover. You can get dressed, and leave whenever you're ready." With that, he walked away and began speaking to the next couple.

A taxi was called and we returned to the apartment, pleased this part of the process was behind us and we could try to make the most of our time in Norway. Emotionally and physically worn out, after a brief chat with my mother-in-law and Isaac, I made my excuses and went to bed, hoping the pain would lessen and tomorrow would be a brighter day.

But the pain didn't subside. It got worse and, although I tried to ignore it, my stomach had started to swell and walking was cumbersome. I had also stopped urinating so often but didn't surmise the seriousness of this. When the clinic phoned me to confirm ten eggs had survived and that they were all doing well, I was relieved. However, following an honest conversation with the nurse about my pain level, she suggested I go to the clinic for a check-up.

I walked into the clinic desperate for good news. An ultrasound confirmed the thirty follicles that had been emptied at the egg collection were now full of fluid that had started to leak into my abdomen. To help alleviate the pain, they carried out an ascitic fluid drainage. This involved inserting a wire guide through a standard IVF needle into my vagina to drain 1.5 liters of fluid to relieve the pressure. The procedure was unpleasant but once complete the pain dulled for a short period. A blood sample was taken and before we left, the specialist confirmed the embryo transfer would not go ahead. Devastated, I tried to blink away the tears that had filled my eyes.

The following day, the 1st of April, I was in agony. The clinic drained a further liter of fluid but this time it was torturous. It took all my strength not to cry out. Because my hemoglobin levels were rising, the clinic admitted me to the hospital. This news sent me into shock. I tried to play it down in my mind, persuading myself that this was just precautionary, and they wanted to be safe rather than sorry.

Once I had gathered my belongings from the apartment, Giles phoned a taxi to drive us both to the local hospital. The building was tall, and the lift ride never-ending to reach the top floor. In the ward, the nurses were expecting me. Tense, I sat on my bed in a room with three other women who seemed to be sicker than me. I felt like a fraud, hated being in the hospital, and couldn't wait to leave. I was sure I'd only be in for one night, and then they'd discharge me so we could enjoy the rest of our time in Norway.

At this stage, the pain was building, and urination continued to be infrequent, no matter how much water I drank. But I was trying to be brave and not cause a fuss. My discomfort was nothing compared to the woman in the bed diagonally opposite me. She was screaming and crying, barely relieved by the pain relief administered through a drip.

Hours passed. I was being ignored, and wondered if I should be there at all. That evening the doctor didn't seem too concerned. He advised me to keep drinking lots of water and authorized a few pain-relief tablets. When my pain increased, I felt as though I shouldn't speak up because the other woman was in agony and still needed a lot of support from the nurses. Visiting hours came to an end and Giles was sent back to our apartment. Hating being left alone, I got ready to settle down for the night, but barely slept. By the morning I congratulated myself on making it through one night and started to pack up my stuff so that I could leave and recuperate back at the apartment. The doctors had other plans.

I was moved to a ward with five other women. The first of many blood tests were taken before I'd eaten breakfast. We waited a few hours for the results during which the pain and swelling around my abdomen intensified. My kidneys were not working properly, and they made little urine. Even though I'd been drinking cups of water, I still barely needed to go to the toilet.

The morning wore on and the pain amplified. I tried to get up and walk around my bed to fetch my iPod to play some soothing music, but I couldn't even do this. I fell back into bed, sobbing with frustration. The painkillers weren't touching the surface. I was close to screaming. Barely able to breathe, let alone talk, my body was gradually filling with more fluid. Just at that moment, my husband, mother-in-law and son walked into the room. They took one look at me and their expressions instantaneously changed from smiles to concern. My mother-in-law looked down with tears in her eyes. She was more than upset or worried–she was scared.

I hadn't gone to the toilet in the past twenty-four hours so I hadn't looked in a mirror. I'd been shielded from my reflection. Giles's mother clearly saw how I felt and understood how sick I was becoming. The fluid was filling my skin which felt tight because of the ever-increasing swelling. My health was rapidly deteriorating hour by hour, yet only my family seemed to notice. *How was this even possible? Where did it all go wrong and why?*

Giles found a nurse, who promptly called a doctor. My breathing was labored, and I couldn't talk properly.

"Hello Sarah, I'm one of the doctors. What's the problem?"

"I'm in so much pain," I sobbed, struggling to communicate through the flood of tears. I crumbled in front of the whole ward, conscious that all eyes were on me. "I can't breathe. I'm scared."

Being stuck in a bed in the middle of the room meant no matter where I turned, someone was observing me. There was no wall to face, no place to hide my fear. The thin curtain around my bed did not mask the sound of my tears or the somber conversation with the doctor. A nurse handed me some tablets to take the edge off the searing pain, and I was advised they would move me to a different room to keep a closer eye on me.

Realizing I was going to be in the hospital longer than we anticipated, Giles returned to the apartment with his mother and Isaac to gather some more of my belongings. While they were gone, the medical team took me to a consulting room to drain the fluid from my abdomen. The room was dreary, and so compact it was almost impractical to fit us all in. Two doctors carried out the procedure while two nurses watched with interest. I lay on a reclining chair with my legs in stirrups, baring all, with no one by my side to hold my hand through the torture. The staff chattered and laughed in Norwegian, every so often speaking to me in

English to explain what was happening. I felt as though I was the freak in a freak show. I wanted to bolt out of the door and banish the pain. But I could barely walk, let alone run. The procedure eventually ended after 1.6 liters of fluid had been drained into a large, metal bowl. Relief washed over my body as the pain eased marginally. Little did I know each time the fluid was drained, it would fill up again and the pain would soar.

My new room was large enough for four patients, but currently empty. I was relieved to have some much-needed solitude to rest until the next patients arrived. A blonde nurse, at least ten years older than me, was calm and reassuring. She spoke little English but enough for her to interpret my needs. The mattress on my bed was changed to a more padded, supportive one, and a metal pan was placed under the toilet seat to begin measuring my urine. She inserted an intravenous drip into the back of my right hand to replace fluid and quickly administer pain relief and drugs to kick-start my kidneys.

That second night sleep escaped me again. I was woken exceedingly early in the morning for my next blood test. It didn't go well. I hadn't drunk or eaten anything. It was like trying to squeeze blood out of a stone. Each blood test stung more than the last and my veins were becoming more elusive. I started to wonder whether there was more going on than they were telling me, but I was too bewildered to ask. When the doctor did his rounds later that day, my worst fear was confirmed.

"How are you?" The doctor's serious demeanor and lack of eye contact made me nervous.

"I'm in a lot of pain, to be honest." I could hardly speak.

"Unfortunately, your body is now dealing with severe overstimulation. We need to keep a closer eye on you. We'll be taking blood more frequently, and you'll be admitted into intensive care shortly."

Shocked and unprepared to hear this, I knew I would not be going home anytime soon. My shortness of breath, low urine production and hyponatremia (electrolyte abnormality) were causing the doctors great concern. Before my IVF treatment started, I knew overstimulation was a potential health risk. But because it affected less than 1 percent of all IVF cycles, I thought the threat would be low. Sadly, this was not the case.

Before going into intensive care, the nurse inserted a catheter, clipping the box to the side of the bed so that my urine production could easily be monitored by the nurses. Thankfully this was the least painful procedure to date. I was relieved that I no longer had to get out of bed to go to the toilet. This simple act had become agonizing. The mere thought of intensive care petrified me. *What if I don't come out?*

I was wheeled in my bed down corridors and in and out of numerous lifts on the way to the intensive care unit (ICU), taking in the startled faces of anyone who saw me. They frightened me even more. Through the doors of ICU, a sea of ghosts stared at me in silence among copious machines, tubes and wires.

Exhausted by having little sleep for some nights now, I foolishly hoped I would have no recollection of the entire nightmare, and wake up when it was over. Being wired up to so many machines and monitors was confronting. The flashing lights, noise and constant ripples of excruciation overstimulated my body and mind. I couldn't get away from it.

Momentarily I felt as though I was back in NICU with Isaac, except this time, I was watching myself through a hazy lens. My own body was attacking me. I was in agony. The drugs made me spacey and out of control as I drifted in and out of restless sleep, waking to nausea and stabbing pain. Through the fog, the chilling sound of machines and monitors reminded me exactly where I was. I rang the bell frequently throughout the night for the nurse to pump more morphine and anti-nausea medication through the IV drip. The relief was quick, and I appreciated those brief moments of peace.

I felt every twinge of pain and wave of sickness as my body deteriorated. The hours dragged by. No visitors were allowed, and there was no TV to pass the time. Not that I felt up to watching anything, even listening to a meditation track was too much. I was ravenous, having not eaten for hours, but no food was provided to patients in ICU. I could only drink water and think. I started to presume other people would believe I had brought it on myself and became convinced that this was true. I wanted to cry, but it was too painful. Those were the most terrifying twenty-four hours of my life.

CHAPTER 10

Would Death Be Less Painful?

Your strength will help you find the light.

O n day four, I left intensive care and was moved back to the ward. In all honesty, I felt no better. My body screamed in agony as though it had been torn from a car wreck. But the worst was yet to come. Each day was filled with intrusive tests, sometimes up to four times a day. I became a pincushion, barely recovering from the last blood test when the next one was due. My arms were bruised beyond recognition through the repeated attempts to locate my veins and swiftly withdraw blood before they collapsed.

The nurses weighed me each morning, measured my stomach and topped me up with morphine and other pain relief. Each time I stood on the scales and saw that my weight had increased, I lost a little more hope. In just a few short days, I had put on a staggering 44 pounds and looked like I was eight or nine months pregnant. Being that large was alien to me. My skin was so tight I felt I might explode. I didn't think my body could expand any more. But it did. I felt unsure whether I could cope or for how long. At the time I didn't register how fundamental hypnotherapy and meditation would be for my recovery. Today I know I would not have got through everything without them.

I underwent one last fluid drainage on the fourth afternoon, but this time I couldn't keep it together any longer. The pain was unbearable. My uterus felt as though it was being shot by sharp needles. "Ow, you're hurting me. Stop!" I shouted at the top of my lungs.

My screams broke the silence. The doctor was stunned by my eruption, unsure why this time it was more painful than the last. Up until this point, I had been so calm, but the hypnotherapy track wasn't working, and my mind was in overdrive.

"Are you okay?" A nurse asked with concern.

"No," I sobbed. "This is torturous. I can't take it anymore."

Morphine didn't dampen the excruciation. Childbirth had been a complete walk in the park compared to this. Reluctantly, the doctor stopped the procedure. He knew only draining 250 milliliters of fluid would not provide my body with any pain relief. I was taken back to the ward by the nurse. On the way, I briefly considered whether death would be better. I just wanted it all to end.

When we entered my room, the nurse told me how worried she was about me. She was much younger than the other nurses, and her warmth and consideration were welcome. I had become such a burden, completely unable to do anything for myself. Vulnerability challenged me like never before. Fiercely independent, I hated being reliant on others for *everything*. I was trying to hold it all together but felt as though I was about to fall apart. The language barrier compromised communication about my health; this left my thoughts spiraling out of control. *What if they are keeping information from me?* The protracted solitude reminded me that we are born alone and die alone. This wasn't the only time I had contemplated my mortality, yet it was the first time I had grasped its full meaning. At times it was too much to bear. In my darkest moments, I suspected the doctors had failed to tell me that I was at risk of dying. Without love from my son and husband, perhaps I would have given up.

I pushed the doctor for more information on the fourth evening. Until now I had been too scared to ask probing questions, unsure whether I was ready to hear the truth.

"The condition should eventually begin to reverse itself," the doctor confirmed. "There's nothing we can do in the meantime except manage the symptoms."

"How long could it take?" I asked.

"We don't know. We need your blood test results to improve and your kidneys are still struggling, which is concerning. When your urine production increases, your weight gain will slow down, which will also reduce the pain. We're going to start administering a drug through your drip to prevent blood clots. We are doing everything we can for you."

Once the doctor had left, I was given my first daily dose of the drug Klexane to prevent thrombosis (formation of blood clots inside the blood vessels). The nurse fought to pull a pair of long white compression stockings over my feet, the nylon somehow stretching around my tree trunks for legs. She unintentionally hurt me but with one last tug, in the end, her persistence paid off. Breathing was still a strain, and I could barely move because of the crippling pain, the stockings doing nothing to alleviate the restriction suffocating my body.

The waiting game continued. Rest was vital, but not forthcoming amid the frequent disturbances for blood tests or checking charts. Desperate for sleep, late in the middle of the fourth night I asked the nurse for a sleeping tablet–a decision I did not make lightly. I cut the pill into pieces. Swallowing them filled me with dread, but concern about the side effects was overridden by my wanting to retain what little sanity I had left. Before the sleeping tablet kicked in, I lay awake, ruminating on the likelihood of us needing to sell our house to pay the hospital bill. As silly as it sounds, we were scared to ask the hospital whether the costs were covered by Norway and Britain's reciprocal health care arrangement, and I needed the medical care regardless. We were also uncertain whether Giles would be asked to go onto unpaid leave and this weighed heavily on our minds. With the mortgage, bills and childcare costs to pay, the longer I was sick, the less supportive and flexible work could be for both of us.

I was often too unwell and tired to talk to or acknowledge my husband, son and mother-in-law's visits. The highlight of each day was Isaac coming up to my bed, full of smiles to see me. Yet cuddling him was intolerable. Neither of us was content with looking at one another across the room, but we had no choice. As much as I wanted to, it was not possible to hide from Isaac how seriously sick I was. On some level he understood. Hospital visits were therefore brief, with me even sadder once he had returned to the apartment.

Isaac had come into the hospital room every day and asked me to go and see the giant teddy bear with him, which lived down the corridor and was the high point of his day. I could barely move on my bed, let alone shift enough to be wheeled down the corridor. Each time I said I couldn't, I watched hurt and confusion stretch across his sweet face. Secretly, I'd made it a milestone to look forward to when my health improved. Now, my motivation was about to leave the country.

The date for our flight back to the UK had crept up on us. Until then we'd thought I'd somehow turn a corner so we could leave Norway together. I was still deteriorating, so we decided that, in spite of the unease caused by a temporary separation, it was best for Isaac to return to the UK with his grandma. Seeing me sick was causing him angst. We felt her caring for Isaac longer term would be much easier in the UK with support from other family members who could amuse him and distract him from what was happening. I was appreciative of my mother-in-law's support and knew Isaac would be in good hands.

Being able to focus on my recovery, with Giles by my side, was a relief. But saying goodbye to Isaac, early on the fifth morning, was not easy. I wasn't sure when, or even if, I would see him again and yet I was unable to hug and kiss him properly. I watched Isaac leave the room for the last time and I started to cry. How I wished things were different.

And then, later that morning, something else hit me with such force. Two or three girls began trickling in and out of my hospital room as day patients, their beds vacated late afternoon, ready for the next girls the following morning. They came with their mothers, sometimes their boyfriends, too, and appeared to be anywhere from about twelve to sixteen years of age. It didn't take long for me to work out why they were there. Memories of my time in the hospital for my D&C procedure haunted me again; I was lying in an abortion clinic for the second time in fourteen months.

The girls laughed and joked with their mothers and boyfriends, seemingly happy and unfazed by their situation. There were no periods of quiet reflection, tears or uncertainty; I'm not sure how I would have coped at their age. As the girls waited for the tablets inserted into their vaginas to take effect, they lay on the bed and playfully passed the time, oblivious to the fat lady lying opposite filled with leaky fluid. When their contractions began in earnest though, they were back and forth to the toilet like a conveyor belt. In the moments when they cried, grasping their mother's or boyfriend's hand, it struck me how young they were. Their cool teenager façades were dropped to reveal their hesitant, girlish faces.

After they left the hospital late in the afternoon, I was finally able to visit the toilet in peace. Opening my bowel was a rare event due to my immobility and deterioration, and one I did not enjoy. It took all my might to get to the bathroom without tripping over my drip stand or disintegrating in a pool of tears because of the sheer effort involved. When I turned the handle on the bathroom door, my eyes were immediately drawn to the toilet. Coated in bright red blood, the toilet was surrounded by spots and puddles splashed on the white tiled floor. Disgusted, I left as hastily as I could, only to see blood splattered all over the ward floor and around the beds. The mess was left for the cleaners to deal with, but not until the following morning. No matter how many times I saw this scene, it upset me. I broke down and cried, only to be abruptly stopped by the physical pain that rose through my body. Even though I had a free schedule to let out all the tears I needed to, I didn't have the energy or emotional capacity to grieve.

That night I pleaded for privacy the next day so that I could recover in peace. As my physical health declined further, I became increasingly self-conscious of my current state and less tolerant of others seeing me like this. On the sixth morning, my heart woke with heaviness as more patients arrived in my room. I reached for the remote control to raise the bed. Through gritted teeth, I carefully moved my legs so that my feet were touching the cold floor, and slowly pushed myself up to standing. With the urine box in one hand and drip stand in the other, I shuffled around the bed, my legs rubbing together, swollen and sore. Drawing the curtains so that I could block out these prying eyes, I only managed to close them halfway.

'Argh!' I screamed. This simple task was proving too much. Crumpling on my bed in agony, I fought to catch my breath, gasping for air through my streaming tears.

Suddenly I became aware of curious eyes staring back at me, evidently alarmed by my outburst. Retreating to the safety of my bed, I dissolved into a quivering, dismal mess. My head toward the wall, I sobbed uncontrollably, the curtain doing nothing to muffle my distress.

One of the mothers stood up and went out into the corridor. Minutes later I heard my name.

"Sarah, what's wrong?" a nurse asked me with concern in her eyes.

"I can't breathe," I explained through tears. "I'm frightened."

"I'll speak to a doctor," she said. "They'll be here shortly."

This was the most testing part of my hospital stay. As a strong woman, I was confronted by what was happening to my body. Petrified, I could see no way out of this.

An hour later I was being pushed in my bed toward the x-ray department, my breathing getting worse. Passers-by frantically averted their searching eyes out of respect for the lady who must have looked as sick as she was. Thankfully, the chest x-ray was relatively painless because I did not have to get out of bed, but I returned to the ward weary. To my dismay the results were unclear; I was sent back to the x-ray department a few hours later. My swollen thighs barely fit the unpadded wheelchair and my body grimaced with every slight bump as we traversed along the draughty, sterile corridors. Repulsed by the sight and odor of the urine box sat on my lap, it was another reminder of what was happening to me. Too weak to be able to hoist this beached whale of a body out of the wheelchair, I was displeased that this procedure needed to be repeated. Once up, I hobbled over to the center of the room where I was asked to stand with my chest firmly pressed against the icy x-ray plate. Horror and anger crept up on me as I questioned whether I could do it. My back hunched over from the excess weight it was carrying, and standing up straight was unbearable. Feeling as though I may fall over any minute, taking a deep breath and then holding it while the x-ray was performed was a real feat. The retest identified I had a moderate amount of pleural fluid on my left lung.

I looked up at the doctor fighting back my tears. No wonder I could barely breathe.

"We are going to administer a drug called Furix immediately. Hopefully, this will be effective, and we can avoid having to drain the fluid from your lung," the doctor advised me. "In the meantime, we will give you some oxygen."

The oxygen mask took the edge off the discomfort, but I was drowning in my own fluid as I struggled to find my breath, any breath. It all became too much. My natural reaction was to cry. To unleash the frustration, pain, and terror. However,

I quickly learned that this hampered every inhale and exhale, and the drowning sensation heightened. My crying stopped as I moved into survival mode and switched off my emotions. Desperate to lie down to calm my body and have some reprieve, I reached for the electronic controller and started to lower the bed. No sooner had I done this, I couldn't breathe at all. As much as I tried to fight it, panic furiously rose in my body as my breathing labored further. With each breath feeling like my last, I was immediately transported back in time to a warm swimming pool in France. I became seven-year-old Sarah submerged under the water, completely out of my depth. Each time I surfaced, I gasped for air before being dragged toward the bottom of the pool again and again. Swallowing copious amounts of water, I began to tire and resign myself to my fate. *Is this how it ends?* And then I felt myself come back into the hospital room, into my breathless body. The controller still in my hand, I had somehow managed to press the right button to steadily raise the bed.

My breathing gradually eased into a more normal rhythm as I got my head around what had just happened. *How have I ended up like this?* A quivering wreck lying in a hospital bed. I was supposed to be on holiday in Norway following a successful IVF cycle, pregnant. My train of thought was interrupted by the nurse bringing me my lunch, a cheese sandwich, and asking me how I was. She could see the strain on my face and following a brief discussion, my oxygen mask was disconnected, and an oxygen tube inserted into my nose. Thankful to now be able to drink, eat and communicate for short periods, I quietly finished my lunch and rolled over to sleep.

Later that afternoon, the same doctor who had administered the Furix drug came back with a colleague and stood at the bottom of my bed with a serious look on his face. Scanning my latest chart, I heard the solemn words, "We're sorry but your chest x-ray shows you have an enlarged heart. We need to send you for further tests–they are ready for you now."

A thousand jumbled questions held my mind hostage. Stunned, I wasn't ready for the answers I might receive so I remained utterly silent. It was as though I was observing a massive wall tumbling down brick by brick without enough hands to catch all the falling pieces. Any attempt was useless as the numerous fragments fell through my fingers. Devastation echoed through every cell of my body. Sitting in the wheelchair, I quietly reprimanded myself as I reflected on my decision to pursue an elective procedure, one that I may spend the rest of my life regretting. *If my heart isn't working correctly, can my body heal? Is time running out?* While these thoughts raced through my head, I prepared myself for more physical torment.

The nurse knocked on the cardiologist's door and wheeled me inside. I was asked to remove my gown and some gel, freezing and sticky, was placed on my chest. The echocardiogram test was savage and seemed to take hours, the ultrasound machine's probe repeatedly pressed firmly against my heart. It was impossible to breathe again; I felt broken. My spirit was beginning to fade; my fear was getting the better of me.

On my way back to the ward I prayed for positive results. I needed something, anything, to be okay. After what seemed like an eternity, I got the best news: no further damage to my heart.

That evening I sat up in bed and briefly spoke to my boss on the phone. We had been exchanging text messages, but now it was time to explain what had happened and that I was unsure when I would be well enough to leave the hospital and return to the UK. She expressed grave concern for my health as I tried to catch my breath and talk properly. It was a difficult call to make because I felt as though I had let my employer down. Due to my personal choices, work was now left to pick up the pieces and pay me sickness benefits during my absence; I felt guilty. Thankfully my boss was exceptionally understanding, and that made all the difference to my emotional well-being and recovery.

During my time in the hospital, Giles was forced to take the vow "in sickness and in health" more seriously than I would have liked. Even though we'd been together nine years, I was embarrassed about the things he was seeing and having to do for me. Giles had been given the unpleasant job of measuring my urine production. But he wasn't run off his feet—there were few measurements to write down.

On the sixth night, I tried to rest my broken body and shattered mind. I thought of Isaac and prayed I would recover to see his beautiful face once more. But beneath my excruciating physical pain, a worse pain speared my heart. A dark fear that I would never hold my son again. It was the lowest point of my life.

***

I thought the agony would never cease, but then finally, on day seven, I began to lose some fluid. My kidneys had a lot of work to do. As the overstimulation process started to reverse itself, Giles took his urine-measuring responsibilities earnestly. His enthusiasm grew whenever he had to empty the urine box. I hadn't expected to see someone so excited about my urine! This made me laugh. I sensed he was pleased to have something to do. Both of us knew that my recovery had begun. The relief I felt was on a par with the first moment I held Isaac in my arms.

Each morning I would wake up to witness urine being slowly pushed the wrong way back up the tubes as the box overflowed. Gradually my blood test results started to improve, which pleased the doctors. My weight gain decreased and, with this, the pain. The monumental strain that had been placed on my back slowly lessened.

Throughout all the drama, I had looked forward to mealtimes. I was always ravenous and eating gave me something else to focus on other than the physical pain. Cheese rolls, salad and apple juice for lunch had never tasted so good, even though it always gave me indigestion. Every day I was presented with the same thing, but I was happy that I was alive to enjoy it. Once I was able to get out of bed, I loved standing at the hospital window. I was thankful to be able to look out to the street below and watch the world go by. I wondered where everyone was going, whether they were happy and what kind of day they were having. These moments provided great solace. They reassured me that despite the whirlwind that was going on around me, of which I had no control, I was still in charge of how I responded. My mind could focus on the uncertainty and pain that lay ahead or gratitude for each second of joy and peace. I chose the latter.

My first shower since arriving at the hospital seven days earlier tested my new mindset. I was so ashamed of how much I smelled that I knew being able to freshen up would drastically improve my mood. But by the time I'd walked to the shower, wheeling my drip and catheter behind me, I was ready to give up.

"I'm not sure I'm up to this. I think I've taken on too much," I moaned.

Giles was by my side. "Sarah, I'll help you. Let's try."

"No, I think it's too soon. It hurts so much. I'm still weak."

"But you'll feel much better," Giles said.

Somehow, I was bold enough to try. Undressing and keeping all the equipment out of the shower was problematic. The extra weight I was carrying meant it was impossible to stand up for long. I also couldn't hold the shower hose and wash at the same time. In the end, I used the shower seat to sit down while Giles gently cleaned my hair and body. The fresh warm water felt so good on my skin, and the aroma of shower gel was a welcome change to the musty smell of urine and body odor. Vulnerability hit me again; I was totally reliant on Giles. I'd never thought that when I was just thirty years old, my husband would need to care for me like this. Despite having seen my body change during my pregnancy and witnessing firsthand all that birth entails, I still wondered whether Giles would look at me differently, without the same love and fondness he once had. As he faced the full magnitude of what had happened to my body, I felt as though I had let him down, particularly so early in our marriage.

In spite of the sizable physical and logistical hurdles that needed to be overcome, with some much-appreciated gentle encouragement from Giles, the shower was completed. With this, I knew I was inching closer to leaving the hospital. I was desperate to return home. I hadn't been separated from my son for more than three days and missed him more than words could explain. I wondered if he felt abandoned and confused, even though he was being cared for by a much-loved family member, and I worried he would be traumatized by what he had witnessed.

In the late afternoon, I eventually managed to visit the giant teddy bear. Sitting in a wheelchair with my trusty drip and catheter, I sat next to the bear, overjoyed that I had made it at long last. Giles took a photo of me to show Isaac when we were all reunited. I was sorry I hadn't been able to go with my son, but this moment reinforced that I was ultimately on the mend. Back in my room, worn out, I climbed into bed to rest and recover. Glancing at the photo of me, I was shocked, not even recognizing the person looking back. *How long will it take to recover?* I realized that after everything I had been through, I would never be the same person, nor did I want to be.

A doctor came into my room that night to speak to me; she was just about to finish her shift.

"How are you, Sarah?"

"I'm all right, thanks—a lot better than I was."

We talked briefly and, just before she left, she gently put her hand on my leg. While looking intently into my eyes, as though she needed to make sure I was listening, she said, "You've been very lucky."

Tears began to well as I understood exactly what I was being told. The doctor looked away. I'm not sure if she was giving me space to pull myself together or whether the glisten in her eyes was because her heart had also been touched. Those words changed my life–they were the beginning of a new chapter, a new life.

Once the doctor left and the hospital noise died down, I lay alone in bed with that conversation playing on repeat in my head. It was a long night, but I was finally able to release the tears, fear and guilt I'd been keeping in so tightly. I sensed the powerful presence of my beloved grandma, her hand in mine. The rings on her fingers felt cold. Her wrinkled skin was opaque but soft due to the swathes of hand lotion she used. How I wished I could see her one last time. Knowing she was keeping me safe brought me comfort and fortitude to get through the night and not give up, no matter what lay ahead.

Throughout my hospital stay, I had a lot of alone time to think about what was happening, and how things could have turned out so differently. The next morning, I replayed my conversation with the doctor to Giles. To my disappointment, he seemed distant, disinterested even. I put it down to tiredness and stress, but also suspected he had not processed the severity of the situation we were still navigating through. I'd had more alone time to do this. Everyone has different coping mechanisms, and sometimes we need space to reflect. At the time though, with all the drugs pumping through my body, Giles's response made me wonder whether I was insane or melodramatic. Nights had always been the worst time for this, while I waited for the sleeping tablets to kick in and drift away from reality. My mind and the constant derogatory chatter were at best empathetic, and at worst judgmental. They had become my closest friends and loyal companions, never leaving my side, even when I was sound asleep. Each night, both in my waking and dream state, I had contemplated whether I would make a full recovery. I observed how deep-rooted my unacknowledged fear about not being able to have another child had been and potentially still was.

Now I had started feeling better and had more energy to face things, I began to fully appreciate what I'd been through. I was grateful that I'd been given a second chance. How blessed I was to be able to reevaluate my life and everything in it before it was too late. The whole experience reinforced that life is a fleeting gift. I knew I was incredibly fortunate to have Isaac, and thankful that Giles had stood by my side during the worst of times. I made a promise to myself, and Isaac, to be the best mom and version of myself I could be. To show him that our mind, body and spirit are connected and that there's so much more to life than our physical reality. I still live by these promises and values today. For this I am proud.

CHAPTER 11

The Long Trip Home

Never give up; you are stronger than you know.

My recovery continued. It was now the 8th of April, 2009, and my eighth day in hospital. I was determined to get out of bed as much as possible and walk around the room to keep the swelling at bay and speed up the fluid loss. This would alleviate the pressure from my back, heart and lungs. My legs were still majorly swollen, brushing together with every movement. I was unsteady on my feet due to the extra weight and having laid in bed for so long. I needed to concentrate not to stumble over the IV drip stand that I dragged around. I was desperate to see Isaac.

At last, later the same day, the moment arrived when I was deemed well enough to leave the hospital and be cared for in the UK by my doctors. This news was completely out of the blue, so we were surprised but ecstatic. Flights and a wheelchair needed to be hastily booked for the following day, suitcases packed, and plans made for Isaac's return home. The hospital's decision had been expedited because a sicker patient had arrived. My nurse had to care for her.

Despite being happy about the prospect of sleeping in my own bed within twenty-four hours, not being jabbed with needles, and allowed to rest in peace, I was also beside myself. Those four hospital walls had become my sanctuary and security. I'd had minimal contact with other people, and I was self-conscious about how ill I looked. I was dreading people congratulating me on my pregnancy, mistaking my swollen stomach for a seven-months-along pregnancy, and then having to explain it was just a large volume of fluid topped with a smattering of trauma.

Fortunately, my mother-in-law had twigged that, due to my weight gain, I would not be able to fit into my clothes, and had considerately left me a pair of her pants. With Giles's help, I managed to pull them up, but could not close the zip. Nor could I tighten the laces on my shoes. My top was squeezed tightly over my fat tummy, exposing my stretched skin. It was not a pretty sight, but I didn't care. I was exhausted and more concerned about how I was going to physically cope with the daunting journey ahead. The nurse removed my catheter, resulting in me needing to empty my bladder every ten minutes. I worried about whether airport queues and rush-hour traffic would mean I wouldn't get to the toilet in time. Giles reassured me everything would be okay.

Regardless of these sobering reminders about how sick I still was, and how slow my recovery could be, I was super excited to be leaving the hospital. At the airport check-in, we picked up my wheelchair and made our way to the gate. Countless rows of inquisitive faces watched Giles repeatedly helping me out of the wheelchair and into the disabled toilet. After the seventh time, I was adamant there could not be any more fluid in my body that needed to escape before we boarded the plane. But I was wrong. With all these eyes on me, I felt a strange combination of embarrassment and amusement. At least I had something to smile about.

The lure of being back home soon was just enough to keep me going through the short, uncomfortable flight. We drove back to Bristol along the country roads, stopping in every village to use the facilities. The massive black cloud hanging over me slowly started to lift as we pulled up outside our house. My heart longed for Isaac and yearned for a proper cuddle with him, but I would have to wait until the following afternoon. Weary, but happy, that night I fell asleep without a sleeping tablet.

"Mommy!" Isaac's little face lit up as he enthusiastically ran into the lounge toward me with outstretched arms and wide eyes.

I hugged him tightly and kissed his delicate cheek. "Darling, I've missed you so much." I smiled. "I went to see the giant teddy bear; do you want to see a picture?"

As I bent down to show him the photo on Giles's phone, he smiled from ear to ear. "Did you like him?"

"I loved him. You were right–he was massive, wasn't he?"

Being reunited with Isaac melted my heart. I vowed to hold him a little bit tighter, for longer and with more tenderness every day.

Over the following weeks and months, we all dealt with what had happened differently. Isaac had understood more about the seriousness of the situation than we had given him credit for. His anguish was revealed through a new phobia of being outside. This was heartbreaking to witness, especially while I was recovering. Isaac recently remarked how sick I had looked, and even years later can still picture the hospital scenes as vividly as I can. Memories do not always fade.

Giles hadn't fully processed what was happening to me while we were in Norway. When we got home, it caught up with him. Giles returned to work and it all came crashing down. He left for work one morning feeling fine but three hours later walked into the lounge and burst into tears. I was taken aback to see Giles so down; he had never been like this before. Giles could now face the fact that he had nearly lost his wife, and that his son could have grown up without his mother. Some counseling through Giles's work helped him verbalize his grief. Giles's boss was so supportive, both during our time in Norway and when we were back in the UK, and for that, we're incredibly thankful.

My recovery was less distressing because I had been able to come to terms with what was happening to me at the time. Hypnotherapy sessions and regular meditation had been fundamental, both before and after the IVF treatment. When I saw my hypnotherapist, she was amazed that I could talk so freely, with little sentiment attached to the whole affair. It was almost as though I was discussing what had happened to someone else, and she felt confident that I was doing well with healing the past. My two sessions under hypnosis took me back to the clinic, the hospital, and the house we had stayed in, resolving anything I was still subconsciously holding on to. I knew in the future I would want to return to Norway to carry out a frozen embryo transfer. This was a safe operation involving no drugs and would be our last chance to have another child. I needed to be able to walk through those clinic doors without angst or unresolved sadness. I needed the transfer to be successful.

Over the following weeks, I continued to attend various medical appointments.

"The hospital must have provided inaccurate results, Sarah," the doctor stated bluntly.

"Why?" I replied with confusion.

"Because these results indicate you were exceptionally sick; they can't be right."

After this particularly confronting moment, I was full of gratitude that I'd recovered and been allowed to return home.

When I raised my intention to return to work with another doctor a few weeks later, she thought I was making the wrong choice.

"Your blood test results show you're still nowhere near back to normal. You'll continue to be exceptionally tired. I'm happy to sign you off for a few more weeks. This will give you time to recuperate."

"It's okay," I replied. "I need something else to concentrate on. I want to be productive again. The longer I'm on sick leave, the harder it'll be to go back."

I was already uneasy about how I would respond to the inevitable questions, and was therefore keen to face people and get this over and done with. I just needed to move forward with my life.

My boss liaised with the university's nurse to facilitate my return-to-work program, which started on the 12th of May, 2009, and personally supported me through my recovery. During this time, my hypnotherapist shared some insight with me that I have not forgotten. She advised me to never let my trauma define me, become my story or take over. Nor to allow this setback to keep me stuck and frozen in time. Because if I did, I risked being unable to fully embrace life. This wisdom was incredibly powerful, and is explored further in Part Two.

To this day, I am still amazed and humbled that I walked away without any long-term health issues. Over time, my body slowly healed from the inside out. At that point, I stopped being hostile toward my body and angry about all the things it didn't do. Instead I started feeling respect and awe. My body had protected me—it had saved my life.

CHAPTER 12

Frozen Embryo Transfer

Hope for new life lies in the freezer.

E ven after everything I had endured, my desire to have a baby never dissi-
pated. All the specialists advised that putting myself through another IVF
cycle would probably kill me. So, this was not something I was prepared to
consider, let alone try. Using our frozen embryos, which had been stored in liquid
nitrogen, was, therefore, our last chance to have another baby. More recently, the
method of freezing embryos underwent some changes. Nowadays, the pregnancy
rate from embryo transfer is much better.[7] But this wasn't the case in 2009; success
rates were lower than using fresh embryos.

Keen to prevent a heart-wrenching decision once our family was complete, I had
never wanted to freeze my embryos. Couples had to choose whether to destroy any
unused embryos, give them to medical science or donate them to an infertile couple.
The idea of killing them felt wasteful and disrespectful. Giving them to science would
have meant they had a purpose and could help others before they were destroyed.
From a scientific standpoint, they were just cells. Yet to me they were potential children—Isaac's brothers and sisters who I would be giving to another family to raise. So
as much as I wanted to demonstrate compassion, and selflessly donate our embryos
to another couple if we didn't need them, I was worried I may not be able to get there.

We had ten viable frozen embryos and wanted to see if implantation could work. Implanting the embryos involved no drugs, and so it was deemed safe; I would never have pursued this if there had been any risk to my health. On the 16th of June, 2009, we flew to Norway and stayed in the same apartment. I did not want to be defeated by what had happened the last time we were there. Keen to rewrite the ending to this tale, facing my fears was an essential part of my healing. As I tentatively opened the bedroom door, I was instantly transported back to memories of me curled up on the bed with a swollen stomach, wretchedly sobbing. Time briefly stood still as though I was reliving that moment. Fortunately, my hypnotherapy immediately kicked in. During my sessions, I had been taught to play this scene on a loop in my mind. Rewinding, fast-forwarding, over and over, until I felt nothing. Thankfully the old feelings did not engulf me. Instead, I became a detached observer, able to put this behind me and refocus on the principal reason for being here.

On the 17th of June, two months after my ordeal, I walked back into the IVF clinic. It felt strange. This place started the procedure that could have cost my family and me absolutely everything. I wasn't triggered though; this was another scene I had extensively worked through until my mind was thoroughly bored of it. I lay on the familiar hospital couch with my legs in stirrups, just as uncomfortable as last time. Two frozen embryos were carefully transferred into my uterus to increase the probability of success. Quick and pain-free, I was grateful that this went smoothly.

Returning to the apartment, I rested, keen to give the embryos chance to implant and develop into a bouncing baby, or two. We excitedly talked about the fact that within the next two weeks I could be pregnant and in only nine months we could be welcoming our second child into our lives. Of course, our enthusiasm was measured. We needed to protect ourselves in case things didn't work out, but this was the closest we'd come to pregnancy for years, and I was optimistic.

Less than two weeks later my hormone levels had increased and nausea set in. I remembered this yucky sensation well. I felt pregnant. Even though it was early, I found the courage to carry out a pregnancy test. Sitting on the toilet, fidgeting with the button on my jeans, two minutes dragged by while I waited for the line to show, or not. Almost too scared to look, eventually I opened my eyes to see a second line slowly appear. I double and triple checked, before rushing downstairs to tell Giles.

I phoned the IVF clinic in Norway to ascertain if it could be a false positive or whether the progesterone, estrogen or ferrous sulfate tablets I was taking may have affected the result. My heart skipped a beat or three when they confirmed I must be pregnant. They also suggested it could be twins as it was early to be showing a positive reading. Wow, now I was really smiling! For as long as I could remember I had dreamed of having twins, and wondered whether my life had transpired like this so that it was now feasible. Maybe the reality of raising two babies at the same time was a far cry from the romantic notion I had created in my head, but that was okay. Even with all the potential costs involved, the practical concerns and being unnerved by the whole prospect, I was still over-joyed. I stood in my bedroom overlooking the picturesque village and pondered everything I had been through to have another baby. It had all been worth it. The loss, the uncertainty, the anxiety and the trauma had finally led me to this moment; to potentially being pregnant with not just one baby, but two. How blessed was I? Ready for the future, I beamed, eternally thankful for another chance to be a mom.

On the 21st of July 2009, we had a dating scan at the hospital, and I was so nervous I felt physically sick. I couldn't bear the thought of not seeing a heartbeat or hearing something was wrong. Again, it felt like an eternity before the sonographer spoke.

"There are two sacs."

I had been right. I would be a mom to twins! But almost as soon as she uttered these heavenly words, I heard, "I'm sorry; only one of the sacs has a heartbeat."

I looked at the screen and could see this was true. Despondency filled me, but then I saw the heartbeat in the second sac and my spirits lifted. Perhaps we could still have a baby, perhaps everything was going to be fine after all.

"There's a heartbeat in the second sac, but the sac is coming away. I'm sorry–you'll probably have a miscarriage and lose them both."

I looked at Giles with despair in my eyes, wanting to deny this was happening again. He looked back at me with such sadness. He was clearly as broken as me.

"Is there any hope?" I whispered.

"There's a small possibility that the heart in the first sac will start beating. But I don't want to get your hopes up. If the second sac remains intact and the heartbeat continues, this may result in a viable pregnancy. I need to be honest though: it's unlikely. I want you to come back next week for a second scan to see if anything changes."

It took a moment for my heart to respond to the news. I didn't want to feel what I knew was coming next, and braced myself for the inevitable sinking feeling. Yet again, I had let Giles down and there would be more pain and grief. I wanted to be swallowed up and spat out somewhere else. *What was I doing wrong?* I just couldn't give us what we dearly wanted.

We went home knowing I had one dead baby inside me, and the other one was barely viable. In the car, we were both silent, preparing for the worst.

Waiting for the next scan was one of the most protracted and desolate weeks of my life. Every niggle in my uterus and every visit to the toilet made me terrified of miscarriage. At the weekend, we drove up to Newcastle, in the northeast of England, for a family christening. At first, I put on a brave face and was grateful for the celebration to distract my mind. But anxiety resurfaced and I reluctantly left the party, unable to keep pretending I was all right when inside I was falling apart. I lay alone in bed crying, resentful of the dead baby inside me. I didn't want it there. But I didn't want the tissue to pass either. This would mean that the pregnancy was over.

The following week, I returned to the hospital and was faced with the news I'd been dreading. The heart had not started beating in the first sac, as expected, and the heartbeat in the second sac had stopped. Even though I'd suspected this was coming, I still wasn't ready for the devastation and loss I felt. I had clung to the 1 percent odds that good news could occur. Yet again, we were right back at the beginning of our quest to have another baby.

The nurse advised that this was another missed miscarriage and with twins, the miscarriage could be particularly distressing and painful. There may be a lot of blood and tissue, two big sacs and many large blood clots. If it didn't fully complete, there was an increased risk of infection, and I would need to go into hospital to have another D&C. So, I made the same choice as last time—the sooner this was done, the better.

Phoning my boss to explain what was happening made everything real. I told her that I needed space to heal and would return to work after I had recovered from the scheduled D&C in a week. I wasn't willing to pass my babies in the toilet at work or on a sanitary towel in a meeting, while I waited for my operation.

In the end, the miscarriage did happen naturally at home, with pain and the loss of a lot of blood and tissue. Passing both the babies' sacs while I sat on the toilet was unpleasant and confronting. They were larger than I had expected. At least I could grieve alone. I cried throughout the day, the depth of my grief continuing to catch me off guard. Sometimes I allowed the tears to flow, other times I resisted them until I no longer could. Whenever I awoke from sleep, the remembering haunted me and caused my heart to crack a little further. My pillow became my confidante, absorbing the copious tears, screams and punches that needed to be set free.

After a few days, I returned to the hospital to check that the miscarriage had completed. It had; surgery was not necessary. Grateful for this, and the heartfelt condolence letter I received from my doctor, I was determined to focus on my future, surrendering to the fact that I may never have another child.

My miscarriage heartbreak and realization that my dream to become a mom again was slipping away were dealt with privately. I grappled to let others in, not wanting to be a burden or potentially compromise friendships. In the past, I had sometimes overshared, shared too frequently or with the wrong people. The disappointment at then being criticized and dismissed, unseen and unheard, was too much to bear again. My natural reaction was to stop being honest about how I was really feeling. I didn't feel safe exposing those parts of myself that I perceived to be flawed. I closed my heart down for protection. Not because I wanted to, but because I needed to prevent further rejection and emotional pain.

On reflection, this wasn't the best way to deal with things. My solution wasn't a sensible one for my mental health and well-being. Imprisoning my own heart only made me more miserable. Instead, I should have been more selective with who I let into my inner sanctum, and only shared all of myself with those I completely trusted. This way, when I needed it the most, the burden of my grief would have been cushioned. It was not until the darkest days were safely behind me that I began to share with others all of what I had gone through trying to have another baby, and the reasons for needing to start a new chapter.

CHAPTER 13

Life Begins in Australia

Listen to your heart and life will naturally unfold.

Starting a new chapter slowly evolved into starting a new life.

Back in January 2008, before we started the IVF process, Giles had been redeployed into the engineering function following the closure of the business development department at the company he worked for. This was a step back in his career and the new role was stressful and unrewarding. The following month, I had my first miscarriage. Disenchanted, I began to reflect on my life. *Why was I feeling deeply unfulfilled? Was there more beyond the monotony of the 9:00 a.m. to 5:00 p.m. existence? If I never held another baby in my arms, would my current life be enough?* Despite knowing I had it all–a divine son, supportive husband, loving families, valued friendships and financial security–something fundamental was still missing. My heart didn't feel full.

The stillness of nature and meditation slowly allowed me to tune into my heart and hear the messages I was ignoring. I share more on how to move out of your head and into your heart in Part Two. My adventurous spirit and desire to explore new countries had been calling me for years. I realized the occasional holiday was no longer enough to quieten my traveler's heart. Every cell in my body pined for Melbourne.

Since returning from China in 2007, Giles and I had frequently discussed emigrating to Australia. However, I had allowed my fear that such a bold decision may not work out, and guilt about leaving my homeland, to overshadow this dream. Our quest to have another child had also taken center stage. But when the recession hit the UK in 2008, and I was still not pregnant, we both knew it was time to stop putting our lives on hold and move forward.

We were hopeful that relocating to Melbourne would enable us to enjoy an outdoors lifestyle and build a better life for Isaac. In May 2008, eleven months before I ended up in intensive care, the visa-process investigation began in earnest. We established that Giles's unexpected redeployment back into engineering was beneficial. Engineering was classed as a critical skill and these visa applications were prioritized. In February 2009, just as we were deciding to go ahead with IVF in Norway, we were able to submit our visa applications. Throughout all the chaos and grief, the Universe was looking after us!

We were on the right trajectory. Only six months later, in August 2009, while I was still pregnant with the twins, our Australian visas were granted. The timing and speed of this approval initially unsettled me. I briefly deliberated about whether it was a wise decision to leave the UK and move to Australia to give birth to the twins, maybe months prematurely. *Would the lack of family support be too much? With no friends to call on, loneliness could be our downfall. Would our unemployment prevent us from being able to access the right health care services?* Despite all these concerns, we set about getting ready to emigrate with a mixture of trepidation and eagerness. In August 2009, Giles and I handed in our notice at work and the eight-week countdown began. Through regular meditation, and sitting in silence and focusing on my breath, I was able to push logic to one side and keep trusting my heart. We couldn't wait!

During this time, I lost both babies. Devastated that once again we were a family of three, I welcomed the extensive to-do list that needed completing before leaving the UK. Being busy helped me to divert my wandering mind away from my grief and onto more positive events. In turn, this sped up the healing process. My focus remained on new beginnings, and the incredible journey we were about to embark on.

Our leaving party was emotional; it became impossible to hold the tears in. I didn't know when we would see everyone again, and hadn't considered that for some it would sadly be the last time. Many people were supportive, others found it difficult to come to terms with our decision. They questioned why we were giving up good careers at the height of the global financial crisis, and knew the substantial relocation costs hindered our return to the UK for at least two years.

Logically, emigrating to Australia made no sense. But in my heart, it did. Learning how to tune into my heart space had developed my intuition. I was willing to follow this guidance, have courage and take the risk.

We are all born with intuition, an innate ability to intuitively perceive and feel. This is the opposite of thinking. Intuition is our internal GPS guiding us through life. Because we are often so busy with day-to-day pursuits though, we may not know how to listen. Consequently, we miss the messages that are constantly being given to help us. Or sometimes, if we are receiving a message we don't want to hear, we may choose to ignore our intuition altogether. Regularly getting still through meditation and connecting with ourselves, or whatever method works for us, means we can feel this guidance more strongly and trust the information that we're receiving. Over time we will take the next step and, importantly, act. If you're keen to develop your intuition, this is covered in Part Two.

Prioritizing our little family and focusing on our happiness was liberating. I was motivated to make the next part of our story successful. On the plane trip to Melbourne in November 2009, I had moments of doubt. As fear crept in, I felt sick about all we'd left behind. I repeatedly quietened my monkey mind through meditation. Bringing my attention back to my breath and reminding myself that I needed to remain open to everything helped me to remain calm. Exploring Australia became my new goal. I persuaded myself that I would have less regret if I gave it a fair go and it didn't work out than not even trying and letting this opportunity pass me by. Mindfulness reminded me to be present and break down each moment into manageable chunks to cope, a priority during both the planning stages of this emigration, as well as the flight over.

We arrived at Melbourne airport in the middle of the night, jet-lagged, yet with enthusiasm and a sense of achievement. From the minute we arrived, I felt as though I had come home. Approaching the Bolte Bridge, we got our first real view of Melbourne, with all the buildings lit up against the night sky. Memories of me crying on the banks of the Yarra River in 2005, reluctant to leave here, flooded my mind. I reminisced about why I had fallen in love with this wonderful city, excited to be sharing this special moment with my husband and three-year-old son.

I took a deep breath, and my body relaxed. My eyes filled with tears of joy as Isaac peered out of the taxi window in amazement. Because we had been brave enough to let go of our old life and trust the Universe, our hearts were fully open to welcome abundance in all forms. The best was still to come.

Life was now in balance. Everything began to fall into place. For the first time, my life flowed. I was no longer in my own way. What does this mean? Subconsciously, or consciously, we can allow our fear, emotions, behavior, patterns and past to stop us from following our true path. Fear is not something we are born with though; it is something we learn from a young age. Our upbringing and environment influences and shapes how fear affects our lives. So, when we learn to walk toward our fears and get out of our own way, we remove these blocks, no longer impede our progress, and naturally reap the benefits. Once I had taken that leap of faith, I understood that life doesn't have to be an uphill battle. I promised myself I would remember this feeling, embrace my future, and continue to make heart-based decisions rather than decisions with my head. Consequently, my life improved with effortless grace.

Through persistence and enthusiasm, Giles managed to secure a job in only six weeks. His success reinforced to me that we had made the right choice. Acquiring a rental property, however, was full of disappointment. Properties were often in terrible condition and prices astronomical. Determined to find a suitable home, I kept asking the Universe to show me the answer.

The tarot was something I had briefly studied just before leaving the UK and, although initially skeptical, the results had continued to intrigue me. While I sat in our serviced apartment searching property listings, I shuffled my cards and asked, 'When will we find our new house?' Immediately drawing the number sixteen, the significance of this was not apparent. Over the next few weeks, I repeated the same exercise twice more. To my surprise, sixteen came up again. What was the likelihood of the same card showing up three times in a row? I knew I must be on to something, but the number sixteen was not making sense. On the 16th of December, 2009, we signed the contract for our new home. We moved in on the 16th of January, 2010, and the house number was 1/15 (1+15=16). I was precisely where I was supposed to be.

It was not fancy but had all we needed. With the beach at the end of our road and the train station next door, Isaac and I amused ourselves with trips to the park and weekly swimming lessons. In a few months, Isaac was due to start four-year-old kindergarten. Vacancies were like gold dust. Undeterred, we put Isaac's name down at a few local centers and left the rest up to the Universe.

While we were on a short trip to Sydney, I received confirmation that Isaac had secured a kindergarten place within walking distance of our house, starting at the end of January 2010! On paper, this turn of events should not have been possible. Once more, I had faith that we were being provided for. All would be well.

Even though I was still coming to terms with losing the twins, I booked an appointment with a fertility specialist two months after arriving in Melbourne. Expecting a six-month wait like in the UK, I was surprised he was available the next month, in January, 2010. I quizzed myself about whether it was too soon, then concluded I would achieve nothing by delaying the appointment. We wanted to ask the consultant whether we could arrange for our eight frozen embryos to be sent from Norway to Australia in the future. We had limited funds to return to Norway any time soon, and the Norwegian IVF clinic was stating that the embryos could not leave the country. Deducing if this was true, and what our options were when we were ready, was paramount emotionally. Hope lay in these tiny, fragile embryos; they were potentially our final chance to conceive.

Before we proceeded with the costly specialist appointment, I took a pregnancy test to rule this out. As expected, it was negative. During our discussion, the consultant reinforced that IVF was not an option because it would likely kill me. Not that I'd have risked putting our family through that again anyway. He was, however, keen to investigate the possibility of flying the frozen embryos to Australia; he didn't want to take no for an answer. In the meantime, I needed to go right back to the basics. I was prescribed drugs to force my body into a more regular cycle and induce ovulation at a specific time. Each morning I took my temperature with a thermometer to detect if an increase in body temperature indicated ovulation was approaching, and updated a chart.

After everything we'd been through, as upsetting as it was, I'd ultimately surrendered to the fact that having another child may not happen. I knew that if the frozen embryos didn't implant successfully in the future, we would be out of options. My focus was firmly on the family I did have, my beautiful son. I was grateful that I was putting my past behind me and starting a new life in Australia. Nobody here knew me or my story. I was no longer the woman who couldn't have another baby; I was Sarah.

On the 16th of January, 2010, we moved to our new house. Later that month, just before Isaac started kindergarten, I discovered I was pregnant—naturally. To say I was shocked was an understatement. With no regular cycle and a body that had not ovulated for years, it seemed nothing short of a miracle. The magic needle in the haystack had somehow been found. We had finally beaten the odds that were so heavily stacked against us.

You'd think I would have been over the moon about this news. And I was. But my heart still felt battered. I was petrified, as it had only been five months since I'd lost the twins. Trusting that this dream could come true for us felt like an insurmountable task; it was the one thing I had spent years wishing for. So, on this day, feeling nauseous and out of sorts, I went through the motions of doing another pregnancy test to quieten my over-zealous mind. As I sat on the toilet with a positive pregnancy result in my hand, I burst into tears. I was filled with dread, as my body was full of drugs that I knew might physically affect my baby's development or odds of survival. I'd already started bleeding and assumed it was only a matter of time before the pregnancy would terminate itself. Bracing myself for yet another miscarriage, I was unable to stop sobbing. I phoned the specialist and talked through the likely outcomes. He tried to persuade me that it should be fine, but as I continued to bleed his words became meaningless. The specialist ordered weekly blood tests through my doctor to monitor my hormone levels. If I was going to miscarry, there was, regrettably, nothing they could do to prevent it. But at least the third time around I was mentally prepared for this, as much as I didn't like it.

Initially, my hormone levels were low and didn't align with the dates I had in my mind. I worried that this was an indication of an unstable pregnancy and for the fourth time I would lose my baby. Nausea and vomiting, or twenty-four seven sickness as I lovingly referred to it, struck me down. But I took this as a positive sign. With each weekly blood test, I was humbled knowing that this increased my chances of cradling a newborn baby in my arms.

Unable to work, still recovering from the significant relocation costs, and with limited income for the foreseeable future, I turned my attention to free activities and entertainment to occupy my mind. Throughout my pregnancy, the local library became my companion. Any spare time was spent reading, which was a real luxury as I had had little inclination in the UK to pick up a book following years of study and a stressful job. Fascinated by self-development, spiritualism and new ways of thinking, I also loved being able to stimulate my mind, which was fading fast under an ocean of hormone changes. My desire for knowledge was insatiable, and my belief grew that we are so much more than our physical bodies. Now I could explore this. That year I visited the Melbourne Mind Body Spirit Festival. My spiritual quest took off as I started enjoying the benefits of living a more curious, intuitive and authentic life. I sensed in my heart that I would be changed for good.

Unluckily, this pregnancy proved just as tricky as all the others. With repeated bleeding, headaches, nausea and dreadful fatigue, I could not dress it up to be anything else. The only peace I got from the sickness and vomiting was when I was fast asleep. But sleeping was not much of an option with a boisterous four-year-old son bounding around needing my nonstop love and attention. By the time I'd dropped Isaac off at kindergarten three times a week, I was ready to crawl back into bed, desperate for any rest I could snatch while he was having fun. In the mornings I couldn't open the fridge without vomiting in the sink. For the first twenty weeks of my pregnancy, I carried a sick bag, a bottle of water and a muesli bar with me wherever I went.

Once twelve weeks passed, I was terrified of having another premature baby in a foreign country without support. The doctors were honest with me that this was a real possibility, particularly as the reason for Isaac's early arrival had never been ascertained. Every week I got through was a bonus.

At seventeen weeks I started having mild contractions and abdominal cramps, just like with Isaac in the days leading up to his delivery at thirty-two weeks. In the early hours of the morning, I could take this uncertainty no more. Luckily, my mother was visiting from the UK, so we were able to leave Isaac with her, fast asleep tucked up in bed. Giles and I drove to the emergency department in silence, terrified I was having a late miscarriage and horrified that, if I were, I would still need to deliver the baby. I lay on the hospital couch while the doctors performed an ultrasound to establish what was happening. After what seemed like an eternity, I was thankfully given the good news that all looked well. This time the silence ended differently. The baby's heart was still beating and the awkward position the baby was lying in was responsible for my discomfort. Giles and I breathed easy and returned home, climbing back into bed to rest before the sun rose.

At twenty weeks, we approached our ultrasound with heaviness. I hadn't wanted to get my hopes up, only to have them come crashing down. To our sheer delight, the scan showed we were having a baby girl, and this time everything looked positive. I didn't know whether to cry tears of joy or scream at the top of my lungs. I'd been shown this cute baby girl in a number of visions some years before, ones I hadn't shared with others because it had felt as though they had been slowly drifting away. Some days I had lost faith that this dream would turn into my idyllic reality. But on the day of the twenty-week scan, I allowed all the nightmares to disappear, and knew everything would be fine.

Isaac was happy that he was soon to be a big brother, although on one occasion he sternly spoke to my stomach and said, "Naughty baby, next time you need to be a boy." Laughing, I believed that once his sister arrived, he would love her regardless. With good signs and some substantial hurdles behind us, I allowed myself to relax, celebrate this pregnancy and look forward to my daughter's birth.

Despite frequent Braxton Hicks around six months, and the doctors being sure I would give birth prematurely, my baby girl managed to stay safely inside until she was thirty-eight weeks old. The night before she was born, I did not sleep a wink. Keen to limit my time in the hospital, I was determined to stay at home for as long as I could manage without any pain medication. As daylight broke, I finally gave in to the contractions and made plans to go to the hospital. An hour later I was stood with Isaac at my friend's front door breathing through a fierce contraction. She had kindly offered to take Isaac to school with her children and then he would come to the hospital at the end of the day to meet his baby sister. The drive to the hospital was only twenty minutes, but it felt like a lifetime.

When I arrived at the delivery suite, the midwife performed a quick examination. She suggested my daughter would easily be born within the next hour as I was progressing so well. She was impressed that I had got to 4 centimeters with just my Transcutaneous Electrical Nerve Stimulation (TENS) machine to cope with the increasing contractions. A TENS machine is a battery-operated device that transmits small electrical pulses to the body to relieve pain. I was grateful for the relief it was providing me now.

The birthing suite felt gloomy, as though it was in a basement, with no natural light or windows to look out of. I didn't like my room and was keen to go upstairs to the maternity ward as soon as possible with my baby girl.

The labor and birth were not straightforward, however. My daughter was lying posterior and numerous efforts to turn her around in the weeks leading up to the birth were not successful. She was having none of it. The pain magnified and I reluctantly asked for some pain medication. Pethidine was injected into my thigh and my labor slowed right down. When I was eventually 10 centimeters dilated and desperate to push, no obstetricians were available to help with the delivery as they were all in the operating room.

"Can I push?" I pleaded with the midwife as she entered the room.

"If you like," she replied. Shuffling some paperwork on the table, she avoided eye contact and promptly walked out.

Does that mean I can, or I can't?

Confused, I decided to breathe through each contraction. By the time the obstetrician had come out of the operating room and was able to assist me, I had started to bleed. My bed was surrounded by a room full of medical staff. Their worry was written all over their faces. With every contraction, my baby girl's heart rate dropped. Time was running out.

Nobody gave me direct instructions and as the pain increased, so did my despair. I just wanted it all to be over. I needed to shut out what was happening to my body to be able to cope, so I closed my eyes and listened to the meditation track I'd used during ICU in Norway. Shortly afterwards, a new midwife with a no-nonsense approach appeared in the birthing suite and promptly took charge. Seemingly more in tune with the seriousness of the situation, she bent down and whispered in my ear, "Your baby is distressed—you need to get her out quickly otherwise you will end up being taken to the operating room for a cesarean."

I shook my head. During the long wait, I'd changed my mind about wanting to push. I just couldn't be bothered and was now quite happy for my baby to stay where she was, despite the indescribable pain. I did not speak or make any noise throughout the delivery, prompting the obstetrician to ask what was wrong with me. He seemed perplexed by my silence. I pressed the TENS machine through the contractions to distract me from the ferocity of my baby's head pushing against my pelvis. Not only was I edgy with the number of people who stood in the room watching me at my most vulnerable, but more seriously, I had started to doubt whether I could do this. The drugs had already worn off and it was too late for an epidural.

"Sarah, this is serious–you're bleeding and need to get your baby out," the midwife reiterated.

I snapped out of it; I had to pull myself together. Drawing on my meditation and hypnotherapy skills, I breathed through the stabbing pains caused by the needle repeatedly pricking my vagina with the anesthetic. I braced myself for what was coming next: an episiotomy. As the obstetrician swiftly cut the opening of my vagina to prevent further tearing and rupture of tissues, pain shot through my insides, causing me to scream out for the first time in hours. With further assistance from the obstetrician and a vacuum, my baby was pulled free at last. Clearly stunned by the birth, my baby was silent. The midwives kept rubbing her delicate skin, trying to elicit a cry. Time stood still. I was in a world of pain and closed my eyes to block out the dazzling lights. Relief flowed through my body as I finally heard a piercing cry; my daughter was okay.

"Congratulations!' the obstetrician announced. "You've had a boy."

A what? I thought, still unable to speak. *A boy? Where is my girl? The one I kept seeing in my dreams. Where's she gone?* But I was in too much pain to voice this confusion. *All the ultrasounds have been wrong. The wardrobe of girl's clothing is now obsolete. At least Isaac will be happy that he has a brother. What are we going to name him?* One of the midwives suddenly laughed loudly and broke my train of thought.

"Can I suggest you have another look?" she said to the obstetrician.

As he did, that wardrobe of clothes was swiftly reinstated. My baby girl, Madison, or Maddie for short, was the most adorable little person I had ever seen. She had a whopping bruise on her forehead, but I didn't care. We instantly locked eyes and I fell in love with her at once. The memory makes me well up whenever I think about it. As I cradled her in my arms, it became clear to me that my miracle baby, who had taken four years to arrive, had been intent on being born in Australia, and her wish had just come true.

The midwives were amazed that I'd managed to deliver her naturally, without ending up in the operating room having an emergency cesarean. Meditation, mindfulness, hypnotherapy and time in Norway had all supported me. At one of the maternal home visits after Madison was born, the same midwife who had whispered in my ear during the birth reminded me that I should be proud of myself because it had been such an intolerable delivery. This feedback certainly explained the physical pain I was still in.

During demanding situations, our minds can help or hinder us. They are our biggest ally or enemy in daily life; we can decide which one. This experience reinforced to me how powerful our minds are and what we're truly capable of, even in our most vulnerable moments. Having the right people around to support us is essential; we don't need to do everything alone. No problem is purely our own, and we forget this. How we think does affect how we feel. I discuss these important topics of mindset and vulnerability further in Part Two.

Four months after Madison was born, Isaac started school. I savored the quality one-on-one time we enjoyed together each day. The baby stage flashed by in an instant and Madison rapidly grew into an energetic, loving toddler. Her white-blonde hair, cheeky sense of humor, and smile that could melt anybody's heart was balanced with her ardent independence and ability to make her presence felt and her wishes known. My heart was full.

CHAPTER 14

The Journey—Life is a Jigsaw Puzzle

It is not until you look back at your life that you see
how every jigsaw piece fitted together perfectly.

I adored being a mom again and felt incredibly blessed to be raising my children in such a beautiful country. After everything I had been through to have Madison, I thought I would be happy to devote all my love and attention toward her while Isaac was at school. However, when Madison was about nine months old, I began to lose myself in motherhood. I aspired for more, desperately wanting a piece of me back. I didn't know what exactly, and felt ashamed for even feeling this. I was scared that doing something for me, no matter how small, would create distance from the loving and funny children I had struggled to conceive and birth.

My soul-searching led me to understand that my heart was longing for spiritual connection to self and other like-minded people, as well as being the best mom possible. I knew it was time to invest energy and money into me. But despite this awareness, the internal conflict with guilt did not subside. I deduced a weekly evening meditation class was a luxury we couldn't afford with another mouth to feed. Perhaps if I ignored this desire, I could silence it. However, when Madison was almost twelve months old, my heart eventually won the battle and

I walked through a local meditation center's door for the first time. The classes were spiritual, and my love affair with meditation continued to bloom. This was my opportunity to understand more about my soul's journey, to connect with my spirit and listen to what it was calling me to do. My self-discovery adventure evolved significantly in 2011; there was no going back.

I read countless self-development and spiritual books. I attended conferences and listened to podcasts, basically doing anything that supported me to open my mind up to new ways of thinking and being. Learning more about energy gradually pushed me out of my left brain, the part responsible for performing tasks that are related to academic activities. I was pulled toward using my right brain more to express my creative side, something my overly analytical mind had previously dismissed. At the time I couldn't have predicted where this new way of being would take me, and how all the jigsaw pieces of my life would fit together in the future. For now, it was just fun.

The more I immersed myself, the more I realized how much there is to life; it's not just a physical affair. Deep down I had always known this. But I had silenced my observations and curiosity for fear that people would think I was mentally unstable.

Growing up, I suppressed my intuition, and pushed aside anything that I could not explain using logic alone. When I was twelve years old, I had a vivid dream showing me that my grandma, my father's mother, was going to die. She had been sick but was now much better, and was being discharged from the hospital the following day. There was no reason to believe anything untoward would happen. I had missed my grandma and couldn't wait to be reunited with her. In the morning, my grandma unexpectedly died as she was being driven out of the hospital gates by my mother's parents. Her final whispered words to my grandpa were, "I feel faint" and she took her last breath.

When I was six, I prayed to the Universe each night for a week that I would become the proud new owner of the year one school tepee. For the past month, we had been able to sit and read a book in this cardboard tent as a reward for good behavior. The exterior had been decorated with our pictures and colorful drawings, and it even had a door that opened and closed. One lucky child out of fifty was going to win this masterpiece. When my name was pulled out of the hat,

I was not surprised. I instinctively knew it was destined to be mine. This was my first experience of the power of our minds and manifestation. Excitedly telling my mother all about it at school pick-up, she was less enthusiastic as she had to carry this unwieldy object all the way home!

My spiritual learnings and new ways of thinking firmly led me to comprehend we're all energy, and each one of us is interrelated. As I reflected further on my life, it became clear I had grown up being extremely sensitive to energy. As a child, I didn't understand what this sixth sense was; it confused me. I assumed everyone could tune into the energy of those around them, but I was wrong.

As a young adult, this continued to perplex me–until I moved to Australia and learned that I'm an empath. Empaths feel deeply and can tap into this energetic awareness. It's an ability that helps us manage relationships, but can also be an affliction when we sense someone is lying to us. Patience is often needed to let the truth unfold. Empaths experience heightened compassion for people, animals and the planet at large, so learning how to shield ourselves and set healthy boundaries is vital. I wish I had understood my sensitivity when I was navigating through infertility. Protecting myself in this way would have made the journey less emotionally painful.

Over the past twelve years, I'm blessed to have met many other empaths, and those who have awakened to the knowledge that something bigger than ourselves is here to support us through our torment if we're brave enough to trust and ask for help. We also all need a tribe. To be surrounded by those who understand and do not judge us. I encourage you to find your tribe as you venture further on your infertility journey; they will pick you up when you most need it.

I was fortunate to have a small tribe around me when my family hit difficulties during Isaac's first year of school. He was an articulate, bright child, but learning to read and completing activities with multiple instructions was not easy. After many medical appointments and a lot of testing, he was diagnosed with dyspraxia. This is a developmental disorder of the brain that causes difficulty in activities requiring coordination and movement due to underdeveloped fine and gross motor skills. It affects every area of life. His sensory processing disorder also led to difficulty concentrating and he was overwhelmed in certain environments. Frustration and despondency became a regular part of daily life for us all. At the same time, it became apparent that Madison had developmental delays. She refused to lie on her tummy and never learned to crawl. Her speech was also delayed. Extensive occupational therapy finally saw Madison walking just before her second birthday, much to our relief. The extent of all the learning differences that Madison was contending with would not be revealed until she was eight years old.

In the meantime, I was desperate to help Isaac and Madison in any way I could. Around the same time, reiki (Japanese energy healing) kept presenting itself to me. I took this as a sign. Increasingly curious about energy, both my own and other people's, I began to study reiki. I was particularly keen for my son to feel calmer, and the benefits of reiki were undeniable. I was intrigued by the messages the body was showing me, and what we energetically reveal to each other without even realizing. Training to be a reiki practitioner was the natural next step. Reiki became a powerful yet gentle way to teach my children and others to tune into themselves and lead more peaceful, fulfilled lives.

In 2012, I began tuning into my intuition more frequently and writing down the guidance I was receiving. Journaling is a wonderful tool. When I recently re-read what I had written, it's uncanny how many things that seemed illogical at the time have since manifested. Journaling allowed me to safely express my feelings and voice my truth. Conveying everything on paper, rather than verbally, was a freeing process. My judgment was not being clouded by other people's opinions or perspectives, which then often inadvertently steered me in the wrong direction. I felt seen and heard. We all need this. I shone a light on my broken parts that needing healing and connected with my heart's desires. As I shifted out of my head and entered the creative zone, my writing revealed that I desperately wanted to try for a third child. Even though this life-changing decision made no logical or financial sense, my soul was urging me to be vulnerable again. To be brave and trust. To know that my fears about having another miscarriage, taking years to conceive, or having a child with developmental delays and learning differences were just that. Fears. Fears that existed in my head. They were not necessarily my reality.

In Part Two, I share some creative journaling exercises to help you get out of your head and deeply connect with yourself. To listen to your sixth sense and receive the intuitive guidance that lies deep inside you, try the "Exercises to Develop Your Intuition" and "What I Need to Know" worksheets. Doing these will enable you to move through infertility, and life generally, with more ease and grace.

After many discussions, Giles and I decided to give ourselves six months to conceive. If we weren't successful, we would enjoy our lives as a family of four. I agreed, desperately hoping that it wouldn't come to that. Identifying that I needed to get out of my own way yet again, I learned to ignore the doubts that would randomly pop into my head. I moved into my heart space and trusted all that was meant to be. Bracing myself for whatever lay in front of me, I was confident that the worst had already happened, and I was ready to deal with whatever was thrown at us.

This time, much to our surprise, there was no delay whatsoever in falling pregnant, even though I was still having irregular cycles. It was as if our baby had been waiting for us to open our hearts and be bold enough to try. Once we had woken up and realized that this is what we wanted, our baby agreed that this is where she belonged. She planned her arrival for Madison's fourth birthday.

As with all my pregnancies, I was back on that rocking boat on the rough ocean. My sickness and nausea lasted for almost five months. Some days I wondered why I'd voluntarily put myself through this again but sought comfort from knowing this would fade into oblivion the minute I held my newborn baby in my arms.

The obstetrician could do nothing to stop my bleeding through the second trimester. It happened for the first time when I was at the cinema with my family. At the end of the film, I went to the toilet. As I sat and looked at my blood-stained underwear, I froze in horror. I feared the worst. That evening I contacted my obstetrician who met me at the hospital and carried out an ultrasound. My heart was in my stomach as I waited for the results. I had lost count of how many silent ultrasounds I'd been subjected to over the years, and prayed for strength to get through the next words spoken.

Thankfully, on this occasion, my baby was fine. I was free to go home, although the obstetrician warned me that if the bleeding carried on, there was no guarantee this pregnancy would continue.

Every day I bled, I prayed that this would not be the start of a late miscarriage. Part of me wanted to shout about my pregnancy from the rooftops. Another part of me knew if I lost my baby, I would be devastated by all the pregnancy comments from well-meaning friends and family. I understand this is a familiar story for so many women, particularly after the first miscarriage. So, on this occasion, I decided to wait until after my twenty-week scan to share the pregnancy news and hoped Isaac and Madison wouldn't spill the beans once they had seen their sibling on the ultrasound. I discovered creative strategies to hide my ever-expanding waistline; fortunately, being able to wear baggy jumpers in the cooler months facilitated this. After twenty-seven weeks, my wish was ultimately granted, and the bleeding stopped. We were through the trickiest stage and the worst was now behind us. Enjoying the remainder of my pregnancy, I began to prepare for the arrival of my youngest child.

At thirty-eight weeks, my labor was, of course, painful. But for the first and last time, I felt in charge of my body and the outcome. Thankfully, my baby was not born two months early, was not lying posterior and did not need to be pulled out in haste. This birth was the most natural and least stressful of them all. My trusty meditation track and TENS machine focused my mind on meeting my child rather than on the pain. By doing this, I was able to remain present and breathe into and through each contraction, rather than trying to push the pain aside. Determined to have no drugs, I relaxed and allowed myself to remember the mantra: "Every contraction takes me closer to meeting my baby." This birth was the final one, and I wanted it to be the way I had longed for the others to be. Proud of myself for honoring my body and laboring without pain relief, the mindset work I had done over the years was instrumental in ensuring this delivery was straightforward and calm.

Baby Grace safely arrived six days before Madison's fourth birthday in a quiet room filled with love and respect. There was no panic, no drama or unnecessary noise. She was peaceful, content and adorable. As I looked into her blue eyes, I felt a deep bond and knew that we had a lifetime of memories to create together. There were also brief moments of sorrow because my soul was acknowledging the completion of another phase of my life. Never again would I experience the joy of discovering I was pregnant. Never again would I wonder what my baby would look like, and never again would I hold a newborn baby in my arms, seeing them looking back at me with the same love I felt right now. So, as I welcomed my daughter into the world, this profound happiness marked the end of a chapter. The conclusion of many years of trauma and debilitating pain, which had also been filled with my brightest rays of sunshine. Appreciation for what I had been shown and learned poured out of me, and I was humbled beyond recognition. The heartbreaking lows and tremendous loss led to the highs, celebrations and joy as I completed not just my family, but also my life.

CHAPTER 15

Dare to Dream Wildly

Limitation resides in the mind. Open your heart, be vulnerable and believe in yourself.

In 2009, my life unraveled like a tightly sprung slinky, gathering momentum as it traversed down steep terrain at full speed. PCOS left a cavernous imprint on me, a tattoo, with its own story to tell. The lowest lows were etched into my core. Broken, I was desperate to banish PCOS or uncover a magic cure. Continually focusing on what was wrong with me, and my failings as a woman, damaged my relationship with myself. At the time, I didn't realize how much. Loving myself was an alien concept. Truth be told, I was still working on liking myself but wasn't doing a good job. Standing in front of the mirror was uncomfortable, fleeting glances were the most I could manage. Peering through the veil of emotion, I saw myself with all my bruises looking back. Each day I rejected myself again, and the little self-worth I had left was slowly chipped away.

While dealing with infertility, I became increasingly disheartened that other people were silent about the one thing that consumed my every waking moment. The isolation I experienced was exacerbated by a lack of understanding, support and inability to talk freely about such a personal issue. Even in a room full of people, I felt alone. Shame got the better of me as I slowly shut down my voice and heart. Disillusioned and angry, frustration and tears came freely and often, but mainly at inopportune times.

On my hardest days, the latest discouraging medical results defeated my spirit. The flame that ignited my core, my soul, slowly dimmed; these were my loneliest moments. I felt as though I needed fixing. But I had no idea where to begin and doubted whether I could even be put back together. There were so many cracks to mend physically, mentally and spiritually before I could accept PCOS and my flawed self. I was eager to be what I considered a "normal" woman but felt disconnected from my body, blaming it for my infertility. I didn't understand how to respect, not criticize, the loving person that existed beneath the bombardment of bad news, pain and trauma. Stress viciously pumped around my body, affecting my mood and ability to make clear decisions. Fear and anxiety were frequently in the driver's seat, obscuring my view. I had not grown up setting boundaries to protect and nurture myself when I was greeted with failure. This unfamiliarity made me feel vulnerable, and I continued to flail around, grappling to understand how to best support myself.

I tried to persuade myself that completing my family with the UK average of 2.4 children was overrated, and that the Universe was doing me a favor. But these attempts were futile. Logic didn't stop the continual ache in my heart for another child. In hindsight, Isaac's conception had been so easy, and I, like many others, had taken this straightforward passage to motherhood for granted. Racked with guilt and inner conflict, I knew I should be content. I had already been blessed with my gorgeous son, while others were still patiently waiting for their first child. But as each fruitless year passed by, and doubt began to set in, the biological urge to feel the heartbeat of a baby on my chest intensified. With every negative pregnancy test and torturous ultrasound scan, I struggled to see a flicker of candlelight at the end of the long, black tunnel. Anything that would provide hope and reassurance to get me through the next inevitable obstruction.

As I reflected on the years leading up to my intensive care admission with severe OHSS and the months of rehabilitation that followed, I realized two things. Firstly, I was being pushed to deeply feel my emotions. Secondly, I survived those chapters due to the unwavering love from those closest to me. I'm grateful for each person who walked alongside me. For those who held my hand, wiped away my tears, carried me, and believed in me when I no longer believed in myself. Their love provided me with the determination and bravery to continue to pick myself up each time I fell.

This self-discovery adventure was indeed raw. Eventually, I got to a point where I had nothing left to lose. It was time to face me–the real me. No longer able to hide behind life's endless distractions, my mindset was reevaluated. Eventually, those periods of darkness were sprinkled with rays of light that became a stunning rainbow, and for that, I am thankful. I understood that each challenge had been offered to me for resolution so that I could finally be who I needed to be. Ultimately finding the strength to walk toward my discomfort, I decided with fierce determination that infertility was not going to define me.

After I recovered from losing the twins, my relationship with my body fundamentally changed; it had to. I became less hostile and disparaging toward myself and acknowledged that self-judgment only makes us feel worse. I grew happier within my own skin. My body had repaired itself so well, despite the immense trauma it had been through, and I finally graciously acknowledged this. I focused my mind on all the amazing things my body did for me, as opposed to the complexities. How it nurtured and supported me in ways I could never have imagined. Stopping the anger and judgment toward PCOS, my body, myself and others allowed me to see everything differently. Resentment softened to gratitude. The happiness and success that I discovered had been lying dormant inside me broke free as my heart started to heal.

If the journey to having my three remarkable children had been smoother, I would still be stuck in my old existence and a life that lacked resonance. As I slowly put myself back together again, I discovered that not only was infertility my biggest blessing disguised as my worst nightmare, but PCOS had ultimately saved my life. Full of thanks for my second chance, I now had an opportunity to cherish my life and change it for the better. For the first time since I was born, I began to accept and love myself, all of me.

Awakening emotionally, mentally and, most crucially, spiritually, I became thankful for the lessons bestowed upon me. Ones that could have taken a whole lifetime to master if I had allowed fear to win. Summoning up the resolve to push myself out of my comfort zone, I released the rope that I had been tightly clutching onto. This led to an extraordinary new life on the other side of the globe, over 10,500 miles from home. The move was exhilarating and the personal growth momentous. My heart opened to receive the most incredible gift, two lovely daughters and sisters to Isaac, that I had almost lost faith in having.

Life was just beginning. When I arrived in Australia, I gained clarity on what I had been searching for since I was a young child. Me. Finding the courage to listen to my heart enabled me to question the essence of who I really was and connect with my why. I understood where my passions lay and what no longer served me. Unsurprisingly, parts of me were replaced with new ways of thinking and being. The mist lifted. I could distinctly see that I had always tried to make the right choices and strived to do my best. It was time to stop beating myself up.

It became ingrained in me that even when I messed up, I needed to have my own back. When I took two paces forward, only to take another three back, I showed myself empathy. This ensured the fall was less brutal, and the marks didn't last as long. Mistakes meant I was closer to success, to being who I needed to be. The tools to build on failure were put into action; I was motivated to keep going. I understood that moving forward didn't always have to be a massive leap of faith, where I felt as though I'd jumped off a mountain with no parachute. Instead, small steps were taken. Any movement sent out a positive message to the Universe that I was ready, willing and able.

This rocky road to motherhood also prepared me for the next unimagined chapter of my life, firmly directing me out of the corporate world. The Universe coaxed me to walk toward my pain, accept change in all areas of my life and find myself in the process. Secondary infertility was the tool that facilitated this much-needed transformation.

With each validation that I was on the right path, I began to follow my intuition more. I learned to feel rather than think, let go of the logic, stop trying to control the outcome and trust. How's that for testing how vulnerable I was willing to be! If I had ignored my inner guidance, I would have missed out on Madison and Grace, whom I can't envisage my life without. All three of my children continue to be my greatest teachers.

Meditation and mindfulness taught me that quiet time for introspection and to recharge our batteries is an imperative part of daily life. We are, after all, human beings, not human doings. Through the natural environment, reiki and expressing my creativity, I was able to get out of my head, move into my heart and be more present. I stopped hunting outside of myself for peace. When I was still, I noticed the space that had always existed between my thoughts, deep inside. There was wonder in simply allowing this peace to be. The noise started to dissipate. This silence enabled me to unearth the root cause of my issues, and, in doing so, evolve–salient components of my metamorphosis. I discovered that even during periods of turbulence and angst, I could still be peaceful and happy, as contradictory as that sounds. I healed from the inside out. So can you.

If you relate to any aspect of my journey, feel alone and wish this wasn't your story, I see you. Infertility leaves many scars. Be gentle with yourself. Opening your heart to healing is like peeling back the intricate layers of an onion. It stings and makes you cry. Each time you remove another layer, one more appears to be healed. Being vulnerable and consciously walking toward your pain, however, will eventually dissolve it. Be courageous and go deeper. Connect with your inner wisdom, your soul, so you can hear and respond to your heartbeat. Choose love for self, not fear. Choose you.

When you're down and stuck on a fairground ride that you can't get off, breathe. You have the key to stop the ride, the knowledge that this will pass. Be kind to yourself while it does. Explore meditation, mindfulness, energy healing and alternative therapies; read books; attend conferences; and listen to podcasts. This will catapult your healing journey and support you to recognize your soul, strength, valor, and inner beauty. You will appreciate that your miraculous body is the only one you have, and that your suffering can be alleviated by adjusting your mindset. The state of your mind and spirit, and how you feel about your body, significantly affect symptoms such as irregular cycles, painful periods, poor sleep, exhaustion, anxiety and depression. PCOS and infertility are about so much more than your body. Your mind, body and spirit are intertwined, and the journey to recognizing this is phenomenal. Part Two of this book guides you through a multitude of ways to embark on a new relationship with your body and yourself so you can heal. Delve in–right now is the perfect time to begin! While reframing PCOS and infertility will minimize the negative impacts on your life, which is needed, also remember these conditions have shaped you into the glorious you reading this book. You are greater than you know. Soon you will know it!

Two of my biggest revelations have been that divine timing influences life, sometimes more than we would like, and impatience never speeds things up. Patience is the ability to accept or tolerate extreme circumstances, problems or suffering without responding with anger, frustration or anxiety. Patience doesn't lessen the pain, rather it cradles it. Being patient through the anguish of infertility and the countless unknowns is excruciating. It's natural to want to escape the pain and ongoing suffering or find a quick fix to avoid the waiting. Letting go of timescales will protect your heart from further pain. I know this is hard. If you are discouraged, are losing hope and want to give up, I send you love. I understand how exhausting it is to stay calm and accept the uncertainty while gracefully keeping the faith for as long as is needed.

Nourish your mind, body and spirit while you wait; the rest is out of your control. Immerse yourself in the great outdoors. Try to shift your worrying thoughts into prioritizing ways to have fun. It sounds counterintuitive, but you need this balance. Joy raises your vibration and softens your heart. As your heart opens, it will attract all kinds of abundance into your life. Joy also makes it easier to believe that your time will come, and brighter days are on their way.

Keep going on this inner exploration until you are authentically you and your most loyal supporter, no matter what. Your self-worth is not measured by your ability to have a child. You are enough. Know that your ideas, dreams, skills and experiences are extraordinary. Get still, often, so you can listen to your heart; it knows what is best for you. Doing this will unlock your future, uncover your calling and reason for being here. One that is unique and perfect for you. Trust that all the answers are inside you. Listen to your intuition and the messages that are continually being presented to you. Doors that were once closed will be opened by the Universe. This will lead to more moments of contentment and improve your chances of welcoming your child into the world. Evoking the flame that silently burns deep inside you will bring forth your passion and motivation to overcome stumbling blocks. Know that you are not reliant on others to pave the way for your happiness and fulfillment; you can co-create your future, and that's exciting!

Through the most meaningful and powerful lessons, I finally let go and surrendered to the Universe and asked for help. This is one of the greatest strengths of all. I learned that everything happens for a reason, even if it makes no sense at the time. As difficult as it is right now to see this, know that the myriad challenges presented to you, and unexpected heartache, also come with benefits. Life is full of duality. Hold onto hope that when your soul is ready to seek them out you'll catch a glimpse. Those experiences that have tested you, and in some cases, even brought you to your knees, will one day be laced with gratitude. It is often in the darkness that we meet ourselves, where we ultimately find the courage to let go and let be. Embrace your jigsaw puzzle, despite the missing pieces. Try to be present rather than focusing on the future so you don't miss the moment you're in. Right now is the only place where you can influence change. Don't waste this opportunity. Once the future does arrive it may not appear how you pictured or hoped it would. But believe that eventually you will look back and see how your pieces fit together, in the right way, at the perfect time. Know that the jigsaw pieces make the puzzle and life you need, not necessarily the one you want. This is the tough and unfair reality of infertility. You can't change it, but how you choose to respond is in your hands. Acceptance will help you to reclaim your power. As you grow through the pain and become your best version, the true potentiality in all areas of your life will be illuminated.

Whatever you are enduring, know you're not alone and there is always hope. Don't remain silent. Please reach out to others. Be vulnerable and speak up. People need to hear you so they can understand the struggles of PCOS and infertility, and how best to support you. Be a voice for those who cannot find theirs, and shine your light. Our truths may be different, but our hearts all beat the same. Sharing your story will help you and others heal. Each of us is a student and teacher. Together we can make a difference in this crazy world.

Show up for yourself and take a step into your new life right now. You are the only person who can do this; it's time! Being brave will change your tomorrow and how this chapter ends. Know you are worthy of happiness, love and abundance, and remember the Universe has your back, always.

Dream wildly!

Part Two

Part Two of this book shares the tools and techniques I used to navigate through PCOS and infertility. These strategies supported me through my darkest moments; I hope they are transformational for you, too. Resources and wisdom are included to help you cope with your pain, trauma and grief. Take your time to work through the activities, and reflect on how you feel. Your emotions will give you clues to what needs healing. The exercises can be repeated often, and will offer different insights each time you do them. My greatest wish is that you embrace the opportunity for personal growth so you can become your best self. Going on this journey will enable you to deeply connect with who you are, deal better with obstacles, and make lifelong positive change.

CHAPTER 16

My Love Affair with Meditation

Delight in silence, connect with your inner truth,
and nurture the peace that already exists within you.

Even though I had read and heard from many people that meditation could help me reduce stress, I resisted it for a few years. Despite the promised benefits, on some level I was dubious about how effective this practice could be. I also convinced myself that it was not the right time. Meditation required financial investment and an ongoing commitment. I already felt overloaded personally and professionally, so learning something new was not a priority at that stage. Procrastination set in. Furthermore, as a recovering perfectionist who lived with a big fear of failure, I worried I may not get meditation "right." I cared too much about what other people would think of me if I didn't meditate correctly, and let the imagined ridicule keep me in my shell. When I reflect, I know these excuses were hiding the fact that I was simply not ready to begin. I hadn't reached a crisis point. Perhaps you can relate to this?

But then over time, my emotions were increasingly difficult to manage. I felt disconnected from my body which I perceived was letting me down. I believed I was failing as a woman. My negative mindset was becoming harder to ignore. As much as I hated to admit it, I knew that work stress, and my building dissatisfaction about not being able to fall pregnant, were counterproductive to helping me conceive. It was this realization that finally motivated me to sign up for my first meditation class.

When I say meditation changed my life, this is no exaggeration. Meditation became the tool that enabled me to stay sane during the craziest of times, and gave me moments of peace when I needed them the most. Meditation helped me deal with the frustrating medical tests and appointments, and the disappointment each month when yet again I was not pregnant. Without meditation, I would not have got through my disastrous IVF cycle. Perhaps I would have become another statistic.

I encourage you to open your heart and mind to meditation, keep reading and persist with this practice in the long term. The benefits of meditation are discussed further in this chapter. As figure 1 highlights, your mind, body, and spirit are completely intertwined. Paying attention to all three aspects of your nature will improve your overall well-being. When you are dealing with PCOS and infertility, it's not just about "fixing" those things that are physically "wrong" with your body. If your mind is agitated, this detrimentally impacts your body and spirit. Perhaps you experience headaches or feel tension in your body. Physical ailments affect your mental health. Then your mental health impacts your motivation to improve the physical issues and relationship you have with your body. It can feel like a vicious cycle. But with the right support, the cycle can be broken. The starting point is simply being willing to try meditation, realizing you have nothing to lose and everything to gain. Because doing whatever you can to keep your mind, body and spirit healthy and balanced is the key to a happy and abundant life.

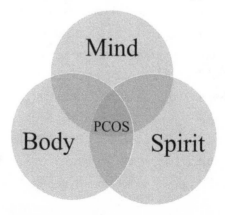

Figure 1: Connection Between PCOS and Our Minds, Bodies, and Spirits

What is Meditation?

Meditation involves completely relaxing your body while keeping your mind conscious or awake. A different state to sleeping, meditation is more restful because it enables total respite. This is hugely beneficial for dealing with infertility, PCOS, and life in general. Your body will thank you for this much-needed pause and quality time for yourself. You will naturally move into this state of deep relaxation when you learn how to observe your thoughts without getting attached to them, release expectations and cease trying to control the process. As you remain open to just being, this space is where the magic unfolds.

According to Dr. Joe Dispenza, an American scientist, author and educator, "if you can continuously move deeper into this state of relaxation while focusing on nothing (or not thinking)—you've just opened the doorway between the conscious and subconscious mind."[8]

Why Meditate?

Research has established that we have approximately 60,000 to 70,000 thoughts in one day. According to Dr. Dispenza, "90% of these thoughts are the exact same thoughts as the day before."[9] This constant and exhausting habitual internal dialogue is lovingly referred to as monkey chatter. When we consider that a large percentage of our thoughts are berating, particularly when life is getting us down, it's not a good place to be. Add the stress and emotional uncertainty of infertility into the mix, and we have a toxic recipe for pain and anguish.

Because many of us don't know how to break this habit, the same patterns and behaviors continue to play out. So it's unsurprising that while our mind regurgitates repetitive thoughts and dramas, the outcomes remain unchanged, and our fertility problems continue. Meditation can help us to change this. The increased space that is created between our thoughts leads to a calmer life. Clarity is attained because our well-versed, wandering, negative mind steals our attention less often. Our capacity to problem-solve grows, and our thoughts become more positive. This leads to us feeling better about ourselves and life, even when the latest pregnancy test comes back negative. Who wouldn't want this reprieve?

Benefits of Meditation

Meditation is different for each person, and, therefore, so too are the benefits. Some people are drawn to meditation for well-being reasons and the promise of improved physical health, more restful sleep, reduced stress and anxiety, and lower blood pressure, to name a few. Meditation also attracts those seeking relief from anger, depression or distress. Others are searching for a more meaningful spiritual connection with themselves, to find their truth, or improve their intuition and decision-making. Regardless of the reason, regular meditation practice facilitates mental, emotional and spiritual growth. All these benefits, therefore, help us enormously on our infertility journey. We are better placed to be able to move our mind, body and spirit into the best state possible to welcome a baby into the world.

According to the Deepak Chopra Center, "new research is also showing that meditation restores the brain. A landmark study conducted by Massachusetts General Hospital found that as little as eight weeks of meditation not only helped people feel calmer but also produced changes in various areas of the brain, including growth in the areas associated with memory, empathy, sense of self, and stress regulation."[10] How exciting to be aware that we can change our brain, that we are not stuck with what we were born with. It is empowering to know that though we cannot control events in our life such as infertility and loss, we are in charge of how we respond. These personal realizations have further deepened my respect and love for meditation.

Benefits of Meditation for PCOS and Infertility

According to Dr. Rebecca Harwin, the PCOS expert, chiropractor and best selling author of *Conquer Your PCOS Naturally*, meditation can support you to lead a PCOS symptom-free life. Meditation can help regulate blood sugar, improve digestion and strengthen the immune system. During meditation, stress, which is known to weaken the immune system, is reduced.[11]

Harley Street Fertility Clinic's director, Dr. Geetha Venkat, confirms that stress has "a negative effect on egg and sperm quality, and on pregnancy rates."[12] Mr. Amin Gafar, medical director at Newlife Fertility Clinic, states that "chronic stress can affect ovulation by altering the hypothalamus functions which controls the release of the hormones responsible for ovulation."[13] Meditating when you're trying to conceive is therefore a beneficial technique to reduce stress. Furthermore, Dr. Venkat explains that "meditation releases another hormone, DHEA, which is known to prolong the life of cells, including eggs."[14] The chance of conception is therefore improved by meditation because the quality of eggs and sperm is directly affected.

Headspace defines anxiety as "a cognitive state connected to an inability to regulate emotions."[15] It can, unfortunately, be common for anyone contending with PCOS and infertility. Dr. Douglas Mennin, anxiety specialist and professor of clinical psychology at CUNY Hunter College, states that "anticipation is at the root of a lot of anxiety"[16] when dealing with infertility, IVF or other fertility treatments. This is because there are ambiguous and unknown elements. "Anything that has high risk and high value, like starting a family, will create anxiety in many people."[17]

Dr. Mennin's advice is that it's important not to ignore your feelings or be consumed by them either. Perhaps you feel as though you are living in a constant state of anxiety? The fight or flight response is an instinctive physiological reaction to a perceived stressful or scary situation. The sympathetic nervous system is activated by the perception of threat. An acute stress response is then triggered that prepares the body to fight or flee.[18] Some of the bodily consequences of the fight or flight response, which you may recognize, are listed below:

1. Thoughts racing.
2. Dizzy or lightheaded.
3. Changes to vision.
4. Dry mouth.
5. Breathing becomes quicker and shallower.
6. Heart beats faster.
7. Adrenal glands release adrenaline.
8. Nausea and 'butterflies' in the stomach.
9. Bladder urgency.
10. Hands get cold.
11. Palms become sweaty.
12. Muscles tense.[19]

Fortunately, meditation can help with anxiety. Research shows that a "consistent meditation practice reprograms neural pathways in the brain and, therefore, improves our ability to regulate emotions."[20]

Meditation also teaches you to acknowledge and process your emotions. Learning how to feel your emotions is crucial when living with infertility so that you can understand and address them. Walk toward your emotions, as confronting as this can be, rather than push these feelings away. Why? Because your emotions will catch up with you in the end, and resistance just delays the inevitable. Doing this also means you'll be able to connect more deeply to yourself and heal much quicker. Releasing emotions from your body so they don't become trapped is much easier when you're being your true self. Meditation helps you to stop fretting about the things you can't alter, of which there are many with infertility, and focus on the things you can. As you notice these changes within yourself, people around you also benefit from your new-found wisdom.

When we consider the emotional side of infertility further, we know that it is common to feel overwhelmed by the desperate longing to have a baby. Impatience, shame, feeling like a victim, and being jealous of other women's pregnancies all show up. As self-love and self-esteem are slowly eroded, arguments with partners, family members and friends can also increase. Tension and conflict in relationships may lead to passionate and sporadic outbursts. Reacting is instinctual, driven by emotions and inner turmoil. Often defensive, the result can be a loss of control.

I understand; I've been there. By focusing on the present moment, meditation helps you respond to others and circumstances, rather than react. Responding contains reason. It's thoughtful, involving a pause and reflection, even if just for a moment. This conscious choice is guided by logic, rather than emotion. Even though it's a more passive approach, responding can alter the course of interaction and is key to living a more harmonious life.

Meditation creates space to allow you to silence the inner critic more frequently, and notice your thoughts about infertility. Your perspective, words and actions can then slowly change. Being more compassionate with yourself and others builds stronger relationships in all areas of your life. In turn, your chances of falling pregnant are improved.

My Experience with Meditation

In the next sections, I share my findings on meditation and what specifically worked for me. Included are tips to get still and different meditation techniques to try, so that you can develop a practice that resonates with you. Meditation doesn't need to be about sitting cross-legged on the floor saying "ohm." Meditation can be fun!

For me personally, my meditation practice began in earnest in 2007 by taking weekly classes at a Buddhist center. Not because I specifically followed the Buddhist philosophies, but because it was a warm, safe place to learn meditation. At the time I was overtaxed at work. My mind was constantly restless with my daily to-do list that never seemed to get done. The stillness relaxed me the minute I walked into the meditation class and kept me returning with enthusiasm. During meditation I felt peace within me, a sensation I had never realized existed. In the early days, this calm was only fleeting, but it made me hungry for more. I longed for the quiet that I previously didn't understand already existed within my mind. Meditation provided freedom between my thoughts, and an inner connectedness that slowly began to shift how I felt about myself. I noticed this silence was different. My mind wasn't held prisoner by exhausting internal dialogue, memories and recycled thoughts playing on repeat. The lightness was akin to floating in the sea without the confines of a physical body, or gliding around the sky with the parachute open after the exhilaration of free fall. At the end of the meditation class, I drifted home happier, more balanced, and carefree.

Regular meditation also positively changed my energy. I felt less overwhelmed and more capable of effectively dealing with what life threw at me. I stopped over-analyzing everything. With my new tools, I was able to face the frustrations of daily life and the highs, lows and stresses of infertility with renewed vigor. Those inevitable tough moments, from which none of us is exempt, still knocked me over but didn't keep me down as long.

The influence meditation has had on my life has been profound. Life can feel like we are standing in a pool of water. Throughout the day each stressful moment, each hurt or failure, is placed into the pool in the form of one cup of water. At first, it's fine; we still have our head above water and can breathe. But as the pool continues to fill up, we eventually need to release some of the water to stop the overload and survive. This is where meditation comes in. Regular meditation lowers the water level, preventing us from getting to that position of sink or swim. It reduces the risk that any cup of water is the one that results in us fighting for breath as our head goes under. Furthermore, being able to keep the water level in our pool at a manageable level changes our perception of life. The indirect benefit of meditation is more joy.

The good news is that meditation is freely accessible to everybody at any time. Meditation has no limitations, and does not divide or discriminate between those who can and those who can't, between those who have and those who do not. In my opinion, it is second only to love in terms of its potential impact on this planet.

How—The Correct Position

Despite the traditional Buddhist meditation notion of sitting in the lotus position on a hard floor for hours at a time, you do not need to sit like this to be able to meditate effectively and reap the benefits. Buddhist monks meditate in uncomfortable positions, or those we perceive to be uncomfortable, so that they learn how to discipline themselves to remain present, while still being aware of their bodies. But they didn't start their practice like this. They built up to it.

The most important thing is that you are physically comfortable when you first start meditating. Otherwise you risk being preoccupied with your discomfort. Keep your spine as straight as you can, with a firm but relaxed posture. Make sure your feet are touching the ground and place your hands in your lap. Sitting in a lounge chair or lying down on the floor or a bed is often not recommended as you risk falling asleep and losing awareness of your body. However, in those instances where this is the only comfortable position, it's better to meditate in this position rather than not at all.

Time of Day

There is a school of thought that advocates meditating at the same time each day to ensure you get into a routine and effectively incorporate this into your life. Setting the alarm and meditating before the house wakes up can work well to start the day relaxed and positive. Alternatively, prioritizing quiet time in the evening will help you unwind and process the day's events before you go to sleep. A routine can ensure meditation becomes a daily habit rather than being a random event that is sporadically remembered during periods of strain or when there is nothing decent to watch on television. But for some people, this routine is not always possible. As long as you don't meditate at a time when you're likely to fall asleep or be preoccupied because you're about to rush out of the door, regular practice is more paramount than when you meditate.

How Long

> *You should sit in meditation for twenty minutes every day—*
> *unless you're too busy. Then you should sit for an hour.*
> (Zen proverb)

When I first learned meditation, I was taught sitting for a minimum of twenty to thirty minutes daily was necessary to reap the benefits. Research and thinking have changed today. According to a study from the University of Waterloo, "just ten minutes of daily mindful meditation can help prevent your mind from wandering and is particularly effective if you tend to have repetitive, anxious thoughts."[21] I have noticed that closing my eyes for just two minutes a day and focusing on my breathing helps me to feel calmer. Committing to this short period of meditation means you enjoy the benefits regularly, start to appreciate the process and are enthused to keep going. It's that simple.

Like any new skill, the more often you meditate, the easier meditation will become. When your daily habit is established, you might start to increase the time you sit each session. This will lead to a deeper state of peace and relaxation that will last for an extended period. The gaps between each thought will become further apart the more you practice. This gives your mind a well-earned rest and is beneficial when you're contending with the stress, anxiety and self-deprecating thoughts that infertility can create. My guided "Breathing Meditation" is nine minutes long and is available to listen to and for download on my website, www.sarahwilloughby.com.au.

Meditation Style

I believe there is a meditation style to suit everyone. Perhaps you consider yourself to be an extrovert and can't think of anything worse than sitting still, quietening your mind and not talking (as expressed by many of my clients over the years). Let me reassure you that you're an ideal candidate for meditation. Working out where to begin and which type of mediation will suit you can be confusing because there are so many options. I suggest reading the choices listed below to find the right fit. Don't worry about doing it "wrong" or getting lost in the "rules" of meditation; just give it a try.

Buddhist meditation taught me to focus on the breath and the sensations associated with my breath moving in and out of my body. I learned how to breathe correctly and that was a revelation. When I mastered this, I moved on to walking meditation and then Loving Kindness meditation. Loving Kindness meditation involves sending compassion and love toward other people and beings. From there I attended spiritual meditation classes where the focus shifted to meeting my spirit guides, receiving messages, and balancing my chakras. I also listened to guided meditations at home. Recently I have been drawn to mantra-based meditations. Today I do a mixture of all these different forms of meditation. My advice to you is to allow yourself to be guided by what appeals to you at any given time. Remain open–there is no right or wrong way to meditate.

Where

If you have access to a quiet, clean room or space in your home, this provides a good opportunity to limit the noise of everyday life. Meditating in the same calm place, even just the corner of a room, triggers your brain to associate this time with relaxation and helps you to settle much faster. Setting up a meditation table creates a focal point for your meditation. Flowers and inspiring images can help instill a sense of serenity in the smallest of areas. Lighting a candle or burning oils can also foster a tranquil atmosphere.

There are plenty of other places to try. Sitting in your car (with the engine switched off), closing your eyes and focusing on your breathing before going into your workplace can be equally useful in creating expansion among the busyness. Locating a quiet park bench at lunchtime and closing your eyes, or playing a meditation recording on public transport can provide the sanctuary you seek. If you're worried about falling asleep, set the alarm on your mobile phone so that you don't miss your stop or an appointment!

If meditating alone does not appeal, research beginner meditation classes near you so that you develop a routine and learn in a supportive environment with like-minded people. Initially, it may be daunting, but you won't look back.

When to Start

In a nutshell, the ideal time to begin meditating and the best place to facilitate this practice already exists right now. It's easy to fall into procrastination, creating conditions and even excuses as to why you shouldn't start in the first place, despite the potential benefits to be realized. If you convince yourself that the perfect circumstances for starting meditation lie just around the corner, you're delaying the start.

It's worth remembering that your future is determined and shaped by your intentions and the decisions you make right now, in this moment. Life will never be exactly how you want it to be. Paradoxically, those times in your life that seem extra chaotic and uncertain, when you don't have the energy to even bother, are when you need to meditate the most.

Be Realistic

Regardless of the ideals surrounding meditation, be realistic from the outset about your meditation practice. Consider what's achievable in your life, including the environment and time you can dedicate to meditating. This means you're more likely to continue and limit the inevitable disenchantment and guilt that comes when you inadvertently set yourself up to "fail." If your mind starts to go there, gently bring yourself back and start again. In meditation, there is no "failing."

Persistence is Key

Even though I have been meditating for years, I sometimes have sessions when I struggle to switch off. If this happens to you, know that it's normal. The key is to not give up. The more you meditate, the more peaceful life will be. "Showing up" and committing to the practice even on low-energy days, and when motivation is lacking, is ironically when the most benefits are realized. Just like after you have exercised, you will be pleased you made the effort.

Connecting to Nature

When infertility was at its most challenging, being outdoors helped keep me sane and enabled me to let go of my emotions. This was one of my favorite things to do because I felt much more peaceful and less stuck in my head.

Have you noticed that you are drawn to go for walks through forests and woods, or on the beach? On a spiritual level, you are connecting to the immense energy of trees, without even perceiving it. The same energetic sensation is realized by observing the sea and listening to the sound of the waves. Each aspect of nature enables you to reenergize from within and brings calm into your life. I encourage you to embrace the great outdoors to help you tune into yourself and self-reflect during periods of stress, grief or anguish. Nature stirs your soul and opens your heart so you can become more loving and compassionate toward yourself and others. Nature is an incredible, free resource to help you work through infertility.

Often our lives are busy and reliant on technology, which leads to our forgetting about the significant physical, emotional, mental and spiritual benefits of being outdoors. Meditating outside and using this as a tool to help us meditate can be powerful. Immersing ourselves in the natural environment may involve a car journey, but it will be worth the trip.

The Beach

This is one of my much-loved places and ways to meditate. Find a quiet spot on a beach, take off your socks and shoes and dig your feet into the sand. Close your eyes while listening to the sound of the ocean. The sound of the waves coming in and out helps to relax you into that meditative state and is exceptionally calming. You can also meditate with your eyes open, and watch the waves rolling out to sea and returning to shore or breaking as they crash against the rocks. This redirects your mind from repetitive thoughts. It's a quick method into relaxation and a simple opportunity to connect with the sea. If you do not live by the beach, listening to a wave meditation while you sit somewhere outside is a good alternative. There are numerous videos of waves rolling onto the beach at sunset and

the sound of the ocean on my Facebook page, Sarah Willoughby Australia. Close
your eyes and relax!

Water

Water is calming and helps you release your emotions. Sitting in a secluded spot
near the sea, a lake, river or pond is particularly peaceful. This enables you to
switch your mind off at the same time as connecting with nature. Try sitting with
your eyes open, breathing in the color of the water with each breath, exhaling all
the stresses and strains of the day.

Swimming is another enjoyable meditation practice. While your body moves
through the water, your mind starts to switch off as you connect with yourself
through your breath and movement.

Listening to and watching flowing water is also therapeutic. If you don't have
access to the outdoors, meditating in the shower for short periods while feeling
the running water on your body, or relaxing in the bath, is also effective.

Walking or Running Meditation—Through a Forest or on the Beach

Walking or running meditations are a lovely means to enjoy Mother Nature and
exercise at the same time—a double win. There is a repetitive natural rhythm that
you tune into when you take a step. Running or walking allows you to be aware
of every movement and how your body feels as it moves. The vibration and sound
of your feet touching the earth naturally helps you to enter a meditative state,
without even having to close your eyes. This method can be tried when walking
or running through a forest, park or on the beach. Notice how you feel as you
breathe in the scent of the trees or the ocean.

Grounding or Earthing

Walking barefoot on grass or sand means you can ground, or earth as it is also
known, at the same time. As each foot touches the earth's surface, you draw the
natural, subtle energy up through the soles of your feet and reenergize. One of
my favorite grounding techniques is walking barefoot on the beach, or in the sea.
As I sense the sand and cool water between my toes, I am truly present in each
moment. I am mindful.

Grounding, or earthing, also helps you move out of your mind, away from "thinking" and the internal noise, and into your body and "feeling." This is the only place you need to be. Your best decisions are made when you are in your body, not your mind.

Meditation for Your Inner Child

Your inner child lives within your psyche. As adults, we often disconnect from this sensitive part of ourselves. We continually seek happiness, believing it is the end destination. In the process, we forget to appreciate the journey and have fun. This leaves us feeling tired, bored, discontent and unfulfilled. When we are connected to our inner child, we feel less stressed and more excited, energetic, joyful, creative and curious about life.

The contentment and simplicity that we enjoyed as a child, of being wholly absorbed in an activity and losing all track of time, is experienced once again. Remaining present and grounded in our body, while also having fun and giving our minds a break from the incessant mental noise, means we are in the present moment; we are mindful. Mindfulness is discussed further in the next chapter.

Other ways to meditate in nature and those that may appeal to your inner child are shared below. If you are blessed to be able to spend time with children, they will also enjoy this quiet time with you.

Sunrise and Sunset

Do you make a concerted effort to properly watch the sunrise or sunset? This is a daily occurrence that we can all make time for occasionally. Is it something you can do today or tomorrow? Maybe it's been so long since you saw this natural display that you've forgotten how it feels. Watching sunrise and sunset in silence can transcend you to that calm place inside of yourself while enjoying the energy of the great outdoors. I encourage you to remain still for as long as possible while you absorb the sky's vast array of colors. If you can't go outside, I invite you to look at some of my videos and photos on my Sarah Willoughby Australia Facebook page.

Connecting with the Full Moon and Stargazing

The moon brings awareness to your inner knowing that you are so much more than your physical body. The full moon is an ideal time to go outdoors and breathe in the energy. The luminescence of the moon reenergizes and cleanses you. Allow the experience to envelop you. The more you look at the night sky, the more you will appreciate the Universe and be reminded of your interrelation with something much bigger than yourself.

Add stargazing on a clear night to your list of ways to connect with the planet and quieten your mind. Just two minutes of staring at the night sky while slowing your breathing can engender feelings of deep peace.

Clouds

Choose a day when the sky is blue and there are plenty of white clouds to observe. Lie on the grass looking at the clouds floating by. This is an interesting approach to meditating and grounding at the same time. Breathe deeply and notice how you feel. You can also stimulate your creativity by observing what shapes and pictures you see in the clouds as they move and change.

Fire

Watching a fire burn and the flames dancing is a wonderful meditation. Observing the flame on a candle is another option if you do not have access to a fireplace or an outdoor fire. Close your eyes and breathe deeply five times. Open your eyes and focus on the fire or flame. The shapes and color of the flames, and the sound of crackling, all add to the sensory experience and ease with which you can still your mind.

Smoke and Steam

Smoke and steam have a similar effect as fire but without the intensity of color. Even standing by a kettle or pan of water and watching the steam as it boils can send you to that quiet place.

Raindrops and Snowflakes

Watching raindrops running down windows or snowflakes falling to the ground through a window are other fun, easy ways to connect with your inner child on those days when you need to stay indoors.

Flowers

Meditating on flowers in your back garden, a park or botanical garden is a beautiful way to connect with nature. Close your eyes, breathe deeply three times and smell their fragrance. Open your eyes, soften your gaze and take in their color. Observe any bees buzzing around them or butterflies flying past.

Be Brave

Meditation, in whatever form resonates with you, helps you deeply connect with self so you can tune into the messages your body is giving you. Change is possible, and this starts with you. Ultimately the shifts you want to make in your life are as significant as you allow them to be. The stillness of meditation helps you move from confusion toward empowerment and positivity. I encourage you to be brave and take a step toward a more fulfilled future. There is no better time to begin meditating than right now!

CHAPTER 17

Be Present, Be Mindful

Yesterday is done and tomorrow may never come.
The present moment is all there is.

Mindfulness combines Buddhism and ancient wisdom of the East with neuroscience and psychology. You learn how to harness the power of the mind through a series of easy skills, purposefully maintaining a gentle and compassionate moment-by-moment awareness of your thoughts, feelings and physical sensations within your body and the surrounding environment. Learning to accept your thoughts and feelings in any given moment, without judgment, is a crucial skill for creating a more positive mindset and compassion for self during infertility.

What is Mindfulness?

Being fully engaged in the present moment with intention naturally moves you out of your wandering, distracted mind and into your body. According to the Breathworks organization, you become "more aware in each moment and step away from habitual, unconscious reactions."[22] This mindfulness practice is developed through teacher-led training, meditation and repeating simple daily exercises, such as the ones I learned below:

1. Brushing your teeth with awareness enables you to notice how the toothbrush feels in your mouth, how the toothpaste tastes and smells, and the noises that are created as you clean your teeth.

2. Eating a meal in silence helps you to taste more and savor the different flavors, rather than being engrossed by what is going on around you.

3. Walking meditation brings awareness to each movement and sensation in your body as your feet touch the ground and your body moves.

4. Regularly taking a minute's break from your computer to focus on an object in the room, disciplines your wandering mind. Pick up your mug or glass. Pay attention to how it feels in your hand: its texture, color, size and temperature.

The Benefits of Mindfulness on PCOS and Infertility

While you are being mindful, your mind is not condemning how your body is behaving. It's not chastising you over why you are not pregnant, or thinking about the next medical appointment and series of invasive tests. Instead, it's enabling you to be fully present, which is the only place to be to positively influence your future.

The increased self-awareness of this state of being also has substantial health benefits, physically and psychologically. Jon Kabat-Zinn, an American professor and author, has been teaching mindfulness since 1979, to ". . . help people cope with stress, pain, anxiety and illness."[23] Additionally, "mindfulness practice has been employed to reduce depression."[24] I learned mindfulness through Breathworks CIC, an international mindfulness organization established in the UK in 2004. Vidyamala Burch, one of the Breathworks founders, trained with Jon Kabat-Zinn so I always felt I was in safe hands.

When I undertook my mindfulness course, I was able to apply what I was being taught to support me through my infertility journey. I learned that pain is not constant; it ebbs and flows. Also breathing into physical pain, rather than pushing it away, softens it. These insights have helped me, over many years, manage the physical pain caused by heavy periods and backache, the physical discomfort of my D&C procedure and miscarriage, and excruciating pain caused by my body's reaction to the IVF cycle. During the course, I met many people who were using mindfulness training as an effective alternative to pain medication.

The Past, Present, and Future

Being present while life occurs means you're not replaying the past. You stop dwelling on all the should-haves, could-haves, maybes or lost chances. Miscarriage can lead to self-analysis and repeated questions about what you could have done differently to change the outcome, and about what would have ensured your pregnancy continued. It can be difficult to move forward from miscarriage. But you must. Please know I say this with love. When you practice mindfulness, you don't miss the moment you're in, because you're no longer focusing on the moment you've just had, and you're kinder to yourself in the process.

If you're contending with infertility, it's common to imagine the worst-case scenario and become absorbed in future worries. Your heart already feels battered. Your mental unease may be driven by loss and past hurts. Conceiving and birthing a baby are such high-reward and high-risk experiences. Living mindfully therefore enables you to be less caught up in a future that often doesn't pan out as you expected or hoped. You no longer waste energy thinking about scenarios that don't eventuate, and creating unnecessary stress for yourself in the meantime. Although you may try to ignore it, your future is not guaranteed; it may never arrive. Right now is all you ever have. This is where your focus needs to be. Being mindful is an easy and compassionate way to improve your mental, physical, emotional and spiritual wellness today, to enhance your tomorrow.

I wish I had understood that my current situation was the leading predictor of how my future was going to look. Understanding this is a game changer. Your future is heavily influenced and shaped by the thoughts you have and the actions you take right now. Doing the same things, and not being present for your life, means nothing changes.

Have you ever thought about how much of your life you've missed because you were physically there but mentally somewhere else? Your mind wanders off and you lose chunks of time. How often have you driven your car but don't remember the route you took because you were on autopilot? Neglecting your thoughts over an extended period means you begin to zone out of your life. Mindfulness can help you to change this, but discipline and practice are required. When I was dealing with infertility, I spent so much time in my head thinking about the baby I was trying to conceive, rather than being fully present to create memories with the beautiful son I treasured. When I reflect on these years, I realize I regularly felt detached, and life passed me by. Fun moments with my son, and being grateful for what I had, were lost. I can't get those moments back. Neither can you. Start now. Make that commitment to yourself to be more present, one moment at a time. Being present gives you the best chance of welcoming a healthy baby into the world. What a gift that would be!

Awareness of Mindful Thoughts about PCOS and Infertility in Daily Life

If you are finding it difficult to train your distracted and critical mind, try asking yourself the following simple questions or reflecting on these statements. These are summarized from a conversation between Kym Campbell, an American health coach, author and PCOS expert, and Judy Robinson, an Australian clinical psychologist.[25]

"Where is my mind currently focused?"

This allows you to notice that your mind has wandered off, so you can gently bring it back with non-judgment to the present moment.

"What's my intention in this situation and the outcome I am hoping for?"

This can be helpful to ask yourself during medical appointments. Even though you will notice judgment exists, and you wish you didn't need to attend consultations or go through intrusive tests, this question brings compassion and kindness toward self. You are also not compounding your feelings by judging the judgment.

"I notice I'm torturing myself" or "I notice I'm wishing."

Noticing your thoughts as thoughts can bring empathy and kindness to them as they take place. These are useful statements to reflect on each month while waiting to find out if you are pregnant. They help you deal with impatience and wanting to know the answer before it's time for this to be revealed.

"I'm noticing my thoughts that I'm a failure. My thoughts don't define who I am."

When you haven't been able to conceive, or have had a miscarriage, your thoughts and feelings can be painful. You may feel guilt or shame or feel like a failure. In these circumstances, it's helpful to consider what you would say to a friend who is expressing these thoughts. What could bring perspective to the situation? What's a caring and sensitive response? These are the words I encourage you to say to yourself during your infertility challenges. When you become self-aware of how you are feeling, you are only dealing with the primary emotion of failure and trying to temper this, not the secondary emotion of anger as well.

"I'm noticing that I'm feeling jealous, and that's a normal emotion."

When your friends or family announce their pregnancies, you may experience feelings of jealousy. But that does not mean that you are your jealousy; you are not a jealous person. Perhaps you then feel guilty about feeling jealous. Naming your emotions is the first step to being able to master them. Reminding yourself that you are not your feelings brings kindness to your infertility experience.

Mindfulness and Social Media

Regularly seeing images and posts of other happy families on social media can be a stark reminder of the very thing that is lacking in your own life. If you let it, social media can act as a negative interference that overloads you and brings you down. I encourage you to limit your scrolling. Mindfulness can support you to keep a more positive mindset, guide your thoughts in a healthier way, and not get drawn into the negativity that can exist in some of these online spaces. I recommend only joining infertility groups and forums that have a supportive vibe. To receive support, tools and tips, I'd love you to join my Facebook group.

Fun Mindful Activities

Play

Play is a valid way to be mindful. When you are playing, you are in the present moment. You are better able to reduce the wanderings of your overly disparaging mind. However, I suspect you rarely permit yourself to play because there are countless "adult tasks" that need attending to first. Play is a vital part of life, regardless of age. Life is serious enough. Dealing with infertility is tough. Just because you suffer through your infertility journey, it doesn't mean you can't also smile or laugh along the way. I wish I'd given myself permission to have more fun, rather than allowing guilt–that I was not pregnant, that I had miscarried our baby, and that I may never be able to give my husband what his heart desired–to overshadow my existence. Simple things like running in the rain, going on a swing at the park or building a sandcastle on the beach can help you connect with your inner child. I particularly like going on rollercoasters and waterslides. Play also helps keep you sane as you deal with your disappointment, loss and grief that the baby you long for has not yet arrived.

Coloring In

Coloring in enables you to get out of your head and connect with more peaceful feelings. It's a fun and cheap pastime that you can do effortlessly. Adult coloring books have been particularly popular over recent years so there are plenty around. I would have benefited from using one in the waiting room before my medical appointments and tests. See if this works for you and helps to reduce your worry and stress.

CHAPTER 18

Creativity and Passion Heal Mind, Body, and Spirit

Creativity is faith and courage to bring imagination alive.

A lbert Einstein stated that "creativity is intelligence having fun."[26] Any form of creative expression that's enjoyable and inspires happiness in your life is beneficial to help balance out the challenges PCOS and infertility present. Creativity takes on many guises, and can be as simple as cooking a meal, renovating a room, painting, making something, writing poetry, singing or dancing. I encourage you to think about how you could express your creativity and what creative endeavors bring you joy.

Benefits of Creativity

I understand that life is busy. Regularly allocating time for these activities and trying new things may appear to be a luxury. You could even feel guilty about spending time on yourself. I know I did after Madison was born. But the joy that creativity cultivates should not be disregarded. As you enter the creative zone and meditative state that naturally develops when you use your brain differently, time seems to stand still, and stress levels are reduced.

Being in a creative flow generates some of your best ideas and solutions to problems. Improving your problem-solving skills will help you overcome the countless blockades that infertility presents. You will also be more receptive to insight that effortlessly comes to you from the cosmic intelligence, the Universe. These are enlightened moments that just feel right. Furthermore, creativity supports self-discovery and strengthens your relationship with self. A vital part of your human experience involves learning who you are, and how your unique skills fit into this weird and wonderful world!

You never know where your suffering will take you, and which doors will open for you at the right time. In the meantime, creativity can provide a sense of fulfillment and joy that will sustain you to cope with infertility: the countless appointments, invasive processes, rigorous schedules and unknown timescales. Fundamentally, creativity will open your heart and prepare your mind, body and spirit to be in the best possible place to welcome a baby into your life.

Creativity Changed My Life

Journaling sparked my creative side and enabled me to switch off my overactive, negative thinking mind. As I became a channel to my own inspiration, I deeply connected with my true self. I realized that all the answers to every problem lay inside me, inside my heart. Writing facilitated loving solutions to rise to the surface, be acknowledged and acted upon. With the materialization of positive results, my anxiety levels reduced.

Safely expressing a previously hidden part of myself was the stepping-stone to spiritual learnings and big life changes. Ones such as moving to a new house in the country by the sea, living my life intuitively, becoming a healer, and coaching others through life's tribulations and infertility. Furthermore, it led to me becoming a number-one international best selling author as a contributor to the third volume of *Business, Life and the Universe*, compiled by Corey Poirier, and writing this book. Trusting my inner guidance to journal also brought me my funny, smart daughter, Grace, and what a blessing she is!

Stimulating Creativity

My creativity is awakened through meditation, yoga, and being immersed in nature. I take photographs to capture the memories and use these in my work to inspire others to go outdoors. Water also allows inspiration and resolutions to problems to surface. Swimming and taking a bath or shower are some of my favorite methods to stimulate my creativity. Washing dishes or boiling the kettle continue to be a quick way to get in the zone so that ideas easily pop into my awareness. Have a think about what could work for you.

Pursue Your Passion

Creativity is also enhanced when you're engrossed in something you are passionate about. Passion reenergizes you and makes you feel alive. For me, exploring new places charges me with excitement about what I will uncover next. The colors, sounds, smells and tastes revitalize my spirit and incite my creative juices. Time escapes me and my heart opens and soars like an eagle taking flight.

What's fun and makes your heart sing? If you had no restrictions, how would you spend your time? What is something powerful that burns intensely inside your core, that inspires you and makes life more enjoyable? When you do what you love, you're energetically filled up and more balanced. Your energy changes and a radiance emanates from within. Others sense this and are attracted to you. As you move into a state of energetic overflow, you have more than enough energy to give to both yourself and others, without depleting your own reserves. Abundance naturally flows; it's the by-product and natural reward that assists the creation of the life you've dreamed of.

I invite you to put aside thirty minutes to complete the "Stimulating Your Creativity" and "What Makes Your Heart Sing?" worksheets. Focusing on your passions helps you learn more about yourself, and takes the pressure off while you wait for your baby to arrive.

Stimulating Your Creativity

This worksheet is designed to help you find activities that will stimulate your creativity. You will need red, orange and green pens/pencils. You may like to copy the table and questions into a notebook. Work through the list and color code your answers for easy visual reference. I hope your willingness to try some of them will be louder than your resistance to being pushed out of your comfort zone or fear of failure.

Red– Zero Interest	Orange– Moderate Interest	Green– High Interest
ACTIVITY		**LEVEL OF INTEREST**
For example: Draw a picture of your house		(RED)
Play a musical instrument		
Take photos in nature		
Make an object out of pottery and paint it		
Play chess		
Write a poem		
Draw a picture of an object in your kitchen		
Make a sculpture out of Play-Doh		
Sit in silence, close your eyes and visualize yourself on holiday		
Bake a cake and decorate it		
Make your dream house out of Lego or building blocks		
Collect sticks, leaves and materials from nature to make your name		
Go to flower-arranging classes		
Draw a picture on your driveway using chalk		
Make a picture out of small crystals		
Create a mood board using Canva		
Write a song		

Make up a short story using the sentence "The purple dragon flew over the haunted house and . . ."	
Do finger painting	
Learn magic tricks	
Make paper planes and decorate them	
Create a necklace or bracelet using colored beads	
Make a dream-catcher	
Plant flowers in your garden	
Make up a dance to show what happened during your day	
Choose a new recipe and make a different dish for dinner	
Paint a picture of something that makes you happy	
Look for pictures in the clouds	
Color in a picture	
Paint stones and decorate your garden with them	
Make a sandcastle on the beach	
Join acting classes	
Make an abstract sculpture from recycled objects	
Date:	© Sarah Willoughby

What Makes Your Heart Sing?

This worksheet can be repeated as often as you like, but ideally every three to six months. Find a pen, a piece of paper and a comfortable, quiet space to sit in. Light a candle and close your eyes for a few minutes. When you feel relaxed, open your eyes and immediately answer question 1. As soon as you have finished writing, focus back on the candle flame for a few moments and then move to question 2. Repeat this process for all eight questions. Do not worry about grammar or spelling. Avoid critiquing your answers. Be open to whatever comes to you and trust the process.

1.   When I'm being creative I . . .
2.   Doing this makes my heart sing . . .
3.   I would like to spend more time . . .
4.   I need to spend less time thinking about . . .
5.   What I need to know right now is . . .
6.   If I felt as though I had no restrictions in life, I would . . .

7. I make the world a better place by . . .

8. My dream is to . . .

Date: © Sarah Willoughby

CHAPTER 19

Get Out of Your Head
and into Your Heart

Trust your intuition: it will always guide you home to yourself.

Gregg Braden[27] is an American author, scientist and international educator who is devoted to bridging science, spirituality and human potential. He has found the heart to be the master to the brain. According to the Heart Math Institute, "the heart is, in fact, a highly complex information-processing center with its own functional brain, commonly called the 'heart brain.' It's an access point to a source of wisdom and intelligence that we can call upon to live our lives with more balance, greater creativity and enhanced intuitive capacities. All of these are important for increasing personal effectiveness, improving health and relationships, and achieving greater fulfillment."[28]

Heart Versus Mind

Your upbringing and schooling have probably taught you to use your mind to make decisions. However, sometimes it can be difficult to quieten the ego, and you get taken down an unfavorable road. Your heart, on the other hand, holds the answers to your problems. Your heart knows the truth. I encourage you to become curious about the messages it is giving you. When you learn to connect deeply with self and tune into your heart and intuition, you will be guided more easily through infertility.

Intuition

Intuition is being able to instinctively understand something without conscious reasoning. When you tap into your intuition, you feel your decisions and trust your gut that something is right or wrong. You interpret what's best for you, even when there is no evidence and it makes no logical sense. Intuition has been helpful in my life to make more accurate decisions quicker; it could be for you too.

The more you use your intuition and strengthen your intuitive muscles, the more your intuition grows. I recommend developing your intuition through fun exercises, such as the ones at the end of this chapter, so that your awareness improves without it feeling laborious. Sometimes you won't be able to see how all the dots joined up in your life until many years later. But with practice and commitment, you will know you are always being steered down the right path, even if it's not apparent at the time. You will trust your intuition implicitly and realize that this inner knowing that comes from your heart will eventually be stronger than any doubt. You won't want to live life any other way.

We don't need to struggle through life alone. Signs and clues to help steer us in the right direction are continually presented to us; they are everywhere. Often we miss the messages that the Universe sends us because we're not present. We're caught up in our head, dwelling on the past or het up about the future. Life is less confusing when we open our hearts and minds to receive guidance, listen to the whisperings of our soul, and ask the Universe to help and meet us halfway. We can co-create our future with confidence!

One of my most memorable moments of receiving guidance from the Universe was in 2007 while watching sunset over Broken Hill, in the outback of New South Wales. The temperature started to drop as the sky slowly turned from a bright blue to an orange-red glow. As the sun set over this vast, stark, dry earth, the sun lowered in the fire-stained sky and the light began to fade. I thanked Mother Nature for this spectacular display and asked for a sign that I was on the right path. A white cloud, shaped like a dove, immediately appeared in the sky above my head, reminding me of the picture on my vision board at home. This reaffirmed I was precisely where I needed to be. Both these photos can be viewed on my website.

I could write a whole book on intuition. It's a fascinating subject and has played such an important role in my life. However, this chapter is just a taster to prompt you to be curious about intuition and invest more time in developing your sixth sense. The worksheet "Exercises to Develop Your Intuition" includes ten simple exercises to get you started. Next, move onto the "What I Need to Know" worksheet to receive further intuitive guidance. I hope you have fun!

Exercises to Develop Your Intuition

You will need a pack of fifty-two playing cards and a small object. These fun games can be repeated regularly. The more often you do them, the faster your intuition will develop. Find a comfortable, quiet space to sit in. Light a candle and close your eyes for a few minutes. When you feel relaxed, open your eyes. See which game you are drawn to. Trust the process. Record your accuracy so you notice your progress throughout the forthcoming weeks/months.

1. Shuffle a pack of cards. Place each card, picture-side facing down, in front of you in four equal rows. Focus your mind on the card/cards you are trying to find listed in exercises a)–d) below. Use your hand to hover over every card and sense when your intuition is telling you to stop. Turn the card over and see if your intuition correctly guided you. Make up your own variations of these exercises:

   a) All the red or black cards.
   b) All the spades, diamonds, clubs or hearts.
   c) Each number seven.
   d) The ace of hearts.

2. Guess what your partner, friend or work colleague will be wearing each day.

3. Advise a friend/family member that you are going to ask them a question that needs a detailed answer. (For example, "Tell me all about the last holiday you went on.") Let them know that when they are talking (for about five minutes) you will go into a daydream state and filter out the words that are being spoken. Keeping your eyes open, you will tune in to what other information comes into your awareness, writing it down so you don't forget. Check afterwards if what you have picked up on is right.

4. Ask someone to hide a small object in your lounge or garden. Try each of these different methods below to see if you can find it.

   a) Go within for a few minutes and ask for guidance to be shown where it is. Notice if you are being drawn to a specific place or area of the room.

   b) Listen carefully and notice if you can hear where your intuition is guiding you to go.

   c) Close your eyes and see if your intuition gives you an image of where the object is in the room.

5. Whenever your phone rings, close your eyes briefly before you answer it, and picture in your mind who is calling.

6. Guess how many emails you have in your inbox each day, and who they are from.

7. Guess who is going to win the sports game or gameshow you are about to watch, and what the score will be.

8. Predict how many red traffic lights you will get stopped at on your drive.

9. Listen to the radio and guess five key words that will be sung in the next song.

10. Ask for the next song that is played on the radio to have a message for you and words you need to hear.

Date: © Sarah Willoughby

What I Need to Know

This activity can be repeated as often as you like, but ideally every three to six months. Find a pen, a piece of paper and a comfortable, quiet space to sit in. Light a candle and close your eyes for a few minutes. When you feel relaxed, open your eyes and read the passage below, imagining that you are there. You may prefer to record the passage on your phone so you can listen to it with your eyes closed and feel yourself in the scene. Immediately begin writing as though the person is talking to you. This person could be somebody you know, someone you have never met or someone who has passed. Do not worry about spelling or grammar, or question what you are writing. Be open to whatever comes to you and trust the process.

The warm sun is shining on your face and you can hear birds singing in the distance. In front of you is a narrow opening leading to a dense forest. The lush, green trees tower above you as you walk along the path toward a wooden bench in a clearing ahead. You notice your name inscribed on a small, metal plaque. You sit down and breathe in the fresh air. Your mind and body slowly begin to relax. You become aware of the sound of running water and see a small river flowing to your left. You turn back and notice a person sat next to you smiling. They say, "Write down my words. It's important you remember them."

Date: © Sarah Willoughby

CHAPTER 20

Be Vulnerable—Surf the Wave of Life

Vulnerability is our greatest strength
disguised as our biggest weakness.

D uring the earlier years of my life, I didn't understand what it meant to feel vulnerable and couldn't label this emotion as such. Vulnerability didn't exist in my vocabulary because it simply wasn't in my awareness. My vulnerability was often masked by anger, frustration and sadness, and was inadvertently pushed aside. To be honest, the topic of vulnerability didn't get much of a look in until I was in my early thirties and I came across a TED Talk titled "The Power of Vulnerability." This talk was delivered by Dr. Brené Brown, American research professor and best selling author on courage, shame, vulnerability and empathy. Watched by over fifty-seven million people, it's one of the most viewed TED talks in the world. I encourage you to check it out.

Dr. Brown explains that "vulnerability sounds like truth and feels like courage. Truth and courage aren't always comfortable, but they're never weakness."[29] I now comprehend that vulnerability is at the heart of all emotions, and when we feel, we are vulnerable.

Because our biological urge to have a child causes us to feel so deeply, being vulnerable seems to be an inevitable part of dealing with PCOS and infertility. This has certainly been my experience. Knowing this doesn't make vulnerability easier to digest, but understanding these feelings are normal helps us to feel less alone.

What I also know to be true is that you can't be vulnerable on this infertility journey without being brave. Your bravery is measured by how vulnerable you are prepared to be. By how many specialist appointments you are willing to attend. How many questions you ask, and second opinions you seek. How many years you keep trying to conceive, despite the emotional and physical pain. How many times you put yourself through yet another intrusive medical procedure, even when the odds are against you. Day after day, month after month, year after year. How many times you breathe through an ultrasound, and pick yourself up after each miscarriage. How much you invest in your dream of having a baby when you know there are no guarantees, and it may not work out. And how long you and your partner can remain positive, despite the repeated bad news, before one of you decides you need to stop trying to conceive.

I know I grappled with my own vulnerability for many years while trying to have all three of my children, though I was unaware vulnerability was what I was specifically facing. Vulnerability for me was remaining calm while waiting to find out whether Isaac had serious complications after his premature birth. Going through IVF was an experience akin to riding a wave that terrified and excited me concurrently. It was an experience that caused great pain, but also provided hope. And a wave that I was determined to keep getting back on until I could take it no more. Vulnerability swooped in as I said my last goodbye to Isaac from my hospital bed in Norway and trusted that all would be well. Lying on the doctor's couch during each ultrasound, excitedly waiting to see my babies' heartbeats, saw vulnerability present itself with silence and then the words "I'm sorry" yet again. Repeatedly picking myself up and believing that one day I would cradle another baby in my arms pushed me firmly into the trenches of vulnerability, only to unexpectedly come out triumphantly the other side some years later.

Dr. Brown established that "those people who fully embrace vulnerability talk about it being necessary, believing that what makes them vulnerable also makes them beautiful."[30] I encourage you to reframe vulnerability in this way.

Grappling with each aspect of the infertility rollercoaster shows your repeated courage, despite how often you might feel weakness and failure. Vulnerability is indeed your greatest strength. I hope you remember this the next time you fall. Know that suffering through infertility is a collective experience, but one that feels isolating because we do not speak about it. Your own vulnerability stories, your dark moments, are ones that are not easy to tell but need to be shared. This will inspire others to do the same.

I invite you to put aside twenty minutes to complete the "Be Vulnerable" worksheet overleaf. This will aid your understanding of your vulnerability around PCOS and infertility. You may be surprised by the insight your responses provide.

Be Vulnerable

Find a pen, a piece of paper and a comfortable, quiet space to sit in. Light a candle and close your eyes for a few minutes. When you feel relaxed, open your eyes and immediately answer question 1. As soon as you have finished writing, focus back on the candle flame for a few moments and then move to question 2. Repeat this process for all five questions. Do not worry about spelling or grammar. Avoid critiquing your answers. Keep writing and be open to whatever comes to you. Trust the process.

1. Do you feel vulnerable living with PCOS and/or infertility? If so, why?

2. Do you allow yourself to be vulnerable, or push your vulnerability aside?

3. How does vulnerability play out in your life?

4. Are you scared to express your emotions and speak your truth? If so, why?

5. Do you prefer to deal with your problems privately and then share them after the event? If so, why?

Date: © Sarah Willoughby

Dr. Brené Brown's extensive research on vulnerability, courage, shame, human connection, authenticity, and empathy has helped me to comprehend more about myself. I've become much kinder to myself through grief and life's messiest moments. As with any emotion and physical pain, leaning into grief, rather than pushing it away, helps to diminish it. If we quash our emotions, they become trapped in our body, stifling us from being our true self and living with authenticity. Unexpressed pain, grief, fear, anger, sadness, and trauma associated with infertility invariably resurface to be healed at a later stage. I encourage you to look at yours. It takes guts to articulate thoughts and feelings out loud; verbalizing is challenging and makes everything real. But with practice, being vulnerable is thankfully less scary. I recommend you follow Dr. Brown's work to help you make sense of your own observations and feelings about being vulnerable. Seek support if needed so you're able to move forward.

Tears are healthy and reduce stress, but we often inadvertently suppress them. Working on vulnerability showed me that I was holding my breath when crying, subconsciously not wanting to feel my pain. Today I allow my tears to flow naturally, and breathe in a normal rhythm when I'm upset so I can feel my emotions and then release them quicker from my body. This will work for you too if you're open to trying it. When I'm low, I also remind myself that emotions are only temporary; they are constantly changing. This five-step process has been helpful in bringing some perspective to my feelings:

1. Acknowledge the emotion.
2. Name the emotion.
3. Observe the emotion without judgment.
4. Gently let the emotion go (crying is encouraged).
5. Repeat.

Life is about duality. Without experiencing deep sadness, we cannot feel profound happiness. Being vulnerable is the only way to embrace life fully. I hope you're encouraged to begin.

CHAPTER 21

Change Your Perspective, Change Your Life

Your thoughts are powerful–use them wisely.

Infertility can feel like a mind game. One that continues to lead to further heartbreak or the ultimate gift. While I was trying to have a second child, I was desperate to cast my negative thoughts aside, but I didn't know how. Swirling around my mind on repeat, my thoughts resulted in so much hurt and made me feel like a failure. Guilt, shame and devastation led to emotional pain that words cannot do justice to. I know you understand what I am trying to explain.

During this period of infertility, I didn't understand that just because I thought something, that didn't mean it was true. I also didn't understand that a thought didn't become more valid the more it popped into my mind. I wish I had known that I could change my thoughts. And that by doing so, it would have also positively changed how I felt about PCOS, my body, and ultimately, myself.

Dr. Wayne Dyer, an internationally renowned American author and speaker in self-development and spiritual growth, helped me understand the power of my thoughts. For this, I am exceedingly grateful. Before he passed in 2015, I was lucky to hear him speak in Melbourne in 2013. One quote deeply resonated with me. "If you change the way you look at things, the things you look at change."[31]

Your thoughts are not fixed, and you are not stuck with them. Because they are transitory, like your emotions, you can change them and tame your mind should you wish. Your thoughts do not define you or make you who you are; you are not your thoughts.

Dr. Joe Dispenza has carried out extensive research into the fields of neuroscience, epigenetics, quantum physics, and the effects of meditation and mindfulness on the brain. His investigations help us to understand how we can rewire our brains, change our thoughts and repair our bodies. When we change the way we think, we can change the way we feel. Dr. Dispenza's research has been instrumental in both bringing awareness to how I felt about PCOS, infertility and myself, and then positively changing this and the relationship I have with my body. I suggest you go to Dr. Dispenza's website[32] to read more about his research.

It's worth doing this inner work because, whether you like it or not, you are stuck with you. The relationship you have with yourself is the most important one you will ever experience; the only one that's guaranteed throughout your life. It's also the longest you have had or will have with anyone. So, it's imperative to make it a good one. This will help you deal better with PCOS and infertility, and feel more positive about yourself. Let's first understand where you are currently at by completing the "Your Thoughts about PCOS/Infertility," "Your Thoughts about Yourself," and "PCOS, Infertility and You Meditation" worksheets. You should set aside about an hour for this process.

Your Thoughts about PCOS/Infertility

Find a pen, a piece of paper and a comfortable, quiet space to sit in. Light a candle and close your eyes for a few minutes. Breathe normally. When you feel relaxed, open your eyes and immediately answer question 1. As soon as you have finished writing, focus back on the candle flame for a few moments and then move to question 2. Do not worry about spelling or grammar. Avoid critiquing your answers. Be open to whatever comes to you. Trust the process.

1. Reflect on your thoughts about PCOS/Infertility. Don't get pulled into a story, simply acknowledge your thoughts and allow the next ones to come. Start to write down all the words. Don't analyze or judge what you are writing, just be honest and keep going. If similar words come up, write them down. Try to push through any resistance that may surface until you have finished. This task may be uncomfortable. It may bring up tears. That's to be expected. Observe how you are feeling, take a deep breath and breathe into your emotions; they are coming up because they need to be released.

2. When you have finished writing, scan the piece of paper and notice the words you frequently use. How many of them have similar meanings? Go through the words and tick those that are positive, then circle those that seem more critical. Ask yourself the following questions:

   a) Were there any surprises in there?
   b) Which words were you not expecting to see?
   c) Were there any positive statements? If so, how many?
   d) Did you realize this is how you felt about PCOS/infertility?
   e) Would you like to change how you feel about PCOS/infertility, accepting that this is part of who you are but does not define you?

Date: © Sarah Willoughby

Your Thoughts about Yourself

Find a pen, a piece of paper and a comfortable, quiet space to sit in. Light a candle and close your eyes for a few minutes. Breathe normally. When you feel relaxed, open your eyes and immediately answer question 1. As soon as you have finished writing, focus back on the candle flame for a few moments and then move to question 2. Do not worry about spelling or grammar. Avoid critiquing your answers. Be open to whatever comes to you. Trust the process.

1. Reflect on your thoughts about you. Don't get pulled into a story, simply acknowledge your thoughts and allow the next ones to come. Start to write down all the words. Don't analyze or judge what you are writing; just be honest and keep going. If similar words come up, write them down. Try to push through any resistance that may surface until you have finished. This task may be uncomfortable. It may bring up tears. That's to be expected. Observe how you are feeling, take a deep breath and breathe into your emotions; they are coming up because they need to be released.

2. Ask yourself the following questions:

    a) Did you expect to see these words? Which ones surprised you?

    b) Is it difficult to see some of those words written down? Why?

    c) Would you dream of saying half those things to someone else? If not, why not?

    d) Have you considered that you are the one person in this world that you should love and nurture the most? If not, why is that?

Date: © Sarah Willoughby

PCOS, Infertility, and You Meditation

I used to think, "If I didn't have PCOS/infertility, I would have more energy, be less hormonal, be able to have a baby . . ." I'm sure you could complete the sentence with your own phrases. When you begin to interrogate your thoughts, your relationship with PCOS/infertility can also shift.

My "PCOS, Infertility, and You Meditation" is designed to move you from your thoughts to your feelings. It can be downloaded from my website meditation store or listened to on my YouTube channel called Infertility—Breaking the Silence.

Find a pen, a piece of paper and a comfortable, quiet space to sit in. Light a candle and close your eyes for a few minutes. Breathe normally. Press play and listen to the meditation. Afterwards write down your experiences and feelings to help you understand more about yourself and your life. Do not worry about spelling or grammar. Avoid critiquing your answers. Be open to whatever comes to you. Trust the process. You can repeat this meditation as often as you feel guided to.

Record your experiences and feelings after listening to the meditation.
Date: © Sarah Willoughby

If you were to do these three activities every day for a week, no doubt you would see that most of your thoughts are rebuking. Successes and self-encouragement are often given far less airtime. This is true for most of us, so please don't be down on yourself and perpetuate the cycle. After all, noticing your thoughts is the first step to changing them, so well done!

Instead, reflect on the criticism you place on yourself and your body, and become curious about how it affects you. By committing to release the past, you can make positive change and allow right now to be the turning point.

Your body will protect and support you through to your final days. I encourage you to tune in and connect with your body; this will help you deal with the unpleasant side effects of PCOS and infertility. I urge you to pledge to be kinder and more nurturing toward yourself, and treat your body with greater compassion. Habits can seem unbreakable. Even when you forget, and disrespect for self creeps back in (and you may not register you do this), try not to judge your behavior. Gently remind yourself that next time you will remember. Do this often, and you will gradually start to see improvements in your relationship with PCOS/infertility, your body, and yourself.

When I committed to this change in thinking and became more mindful of my thoughts, my symptoms and the impact they had on my life were reduced. My periods became lighter, not so painful, and less erratic. I began forcing myself to look into my own eyes in the mirror and say, "Sarah, I love you. I really love you." At first, I cringed. But I persisted until I no longer winced and looked away, until I believed what I was saying. Doing this helped me to connect with my soul and acknowledge the person looking back who needed more love, compassion and kindness, not criticism. From this point forward PCOS and infertility became fragments of myself that I learned to accept, rather than disown. They did not solely define me. I no longer gave them this power; I hope in time you can do the same. Perhaps you are skeptical about changing the way you think to change the way you feel? If so, ask yourself what have you got to lose? Most of our thoughts are repeated anyway—you might not miss a few of the less-positive ones.

I hope the exercises in this chapter help you to come to that place of acceptance, because when you change your perspective, everything changes. It really is as easy and as hard as that. I know this is a confusing contradiction.

Over many years of reading books, investing in my personal growth and discussing life with others, I have grappled with the prospect that our perceptions about ourselves and others are not reality. It was thought-provoking to learn that all we surmise to be true is just an illusion. It led me to ask myself, if I am not my thoughts and beliefs, then *Who am I?* As I discarded the labels I and others had given me over the years, it became clear that I didn't know. Removing the titles of mother, sister, daughter, friend, business owner, coach, healer and so on, left me contemplating what remained.

The label "infertile woman" that I had carried for so long, emblazoned on my heart like a badge of honor, had done so much damage to my psyche and confidence. The irony was that "infertile" was not who I was, or who you are. You are not "infertility warrior" or "PCOS fighter," "PCOS sufferer" or "infertility survivor." You are not any of your labels. You are so much more.

Sadly, most of us don't truly know who we are because we allow people's opinions to unduly influence us. You aren't the expectations others place on you. Nor the stories they have created for you or about you. Ones that you subconsciously adopt as your own. When you know that it's none of your business what others think of you, you'll be liberated to live life as yourself. And doing so makes your infertility journey so much easier.

We often don't give ourselves quality time because we are taught to put others' needs before our own. Our sacred relationship with self is neglected. When we give all of ourselves to others, we have nothing left for us. Like fitting an oxygen mask on a plane, the risk is, we could die while caring for someone else. We must understand ourselves because this is our birthright. It also has an incredible ripple effect on those around us; everybody wins!

Asking the question, "Who am I?" is the most confronting one you will ever ask yourself. In my experience, and from working extensively with others, unless you know the answer to this question, you will continue to seek temporary happiness from material possessions, relationships, people and places. Unfortunately, these external things will not be enough to satisfy you in the long term, and your soul will always crave deeper fulfillment.

I invite you to sit quietly and allow your soul to rise, so that you begin to recognize that you are neither the thoughts and opinions you or others have about yourself, nor your labels or roles. Let's spend twenty minutes working through the "Who Am I?" worksheet now.

Who Am I?

When you allow yourself to connect with your soul, at the core, you will discover the essence of who you are and what you yearn for. Find a pen, a piece of paper and a comfortable, quiet space to sit. Light a candle and close your eyes for a few minutes. When you feel relaxed, open your eyes and immediately answer question 1. As soon as you have finished writing, focus back on the candle flame for a few moments and then move to question 2. Do not worry about spelling or grammar. Avoid critiquing your answers. Be open to whatever comes to you. Trust the process.

If you are comfortable doing so, talk to close friends or family. Ask them who they see you as. You may be surprised by the responses you receive. This could help you to understand aspects of yourself that you weren't aware of or were previously hidden. But remember to never take on others' insight that doesn't resonate with you.

---

1. Remove the roles you play. Sister, wife, daughter, mother, friend, employee, employer, colleague, mentor, neighbor or anything else you have labeled yourself to be. Take away your positions, responsibilities, health situation and personal appearance. Repeat gently, "Who am I?" over and over until the noise dissipates and you begin to hear the whisperings of your own heart.

2. Ask yourself: "What do I desire?" The answers may surprise you, or silence may greet you. Cast aside the limitations you place on yourself. What are you left with?

Date: © Sarah Willoughby

After initially removing all your cloaks of protection, like me, you may be left naked and exposed, with no idea how to put yourself back together again. I spent over twelve months embracing my vulnerability and ruminating further on who I was. Recording my dreams in a journal provided insight into which areas of my life I was struggling with. Regularly writing down how I was feeling, even when my thoughts were irrational, helped me through this confusing period. The journaling process allowed me to be honest with myself about what I needed to change in my life to manage my PCOS symptoms better and feel more vibrant. I then acted in the following ways, which may also improve your experience with infertility:

1. I became more mindful of what I was putting into my body. I increased my intake of fresh food and drank less alcohol.
2. I reduced my caffeine intake. This was easy for me as I don't like coffee and tea, but I tried to eat less chocolate. I am still working on this!
3. I increased my water intake which made me feel less tired. I had previously been unaware how frequently I was dehydrated, only drinking when I was thirsty rather than continuously throughout the day.
4. I worked with a personal trainer and got fit. This helped me to deal with the fluctuations in hormones and mood swings.
5. I swam regularly to feel more balanced.
6. I spent time in my garden every day to ground and connect with the great outdoors.
7. I walked in nature to breathe properly and still my mind. My energy instantly changed as I moved out of my overactive mind with my negative thoughts and into my body.
8. I meditated every day and practiced mindfulness to be more present in my life and repair my relationship with self.
9. I connected regularly with my tribe to keep me accountable for my ongoing personal growth and more positive mindset.
10. I gave myself reiki to acknowledge and release blockages in my energy.
11. I practiced self-care every day so I could recharge before I burned out.
12. I took up yoga to connect with my true self and deal better with life's trials.

Kirsty Saunders, an Australian yoga teacher, meditation and energy guide, has been such a blessing in my and my children's lives. Kirsty has an online yoga studio and meditation hub so you can learn in the comfort of your own home. I highly recommend you connect with Kirsty via her website[33] to understand how she can enhance your well-being.

Doing these things has specifically improved my well-being, though I strongly advise you to seek the relevant medical advice for yourself because we are all different.

Affirmations

Noticing your negative thoughts about yourself is the first strategy to becoming less disapproving of yourself. Affirmations help you to interrupt your thought patterns and, in time, look at situations and yourself from a different angle. Say each affirmation, such as the ones listed below, three times out loud regularly throughout the day. Use reminders to help you to remember to say them, such as every time you boil the kettle or sit at a red traffic light. Keep going until you sense that subtle energetic shift and believe what you're saying. In time you will feel you are enough just the way you are.

1. "I am enough."
2. "I am love."
3. "I have everything I need."

Altering your frame of reference so that you accept nothing is either "good" or "bad," also means that your experiences alter, and life begins to transpire differently. If you feel you are losing hope of having a baby and begin slipping into thoughts of "why me?", try turning it around to "why not me?" Feel the energetic shift and empowerment that comes from this subtle reframing. The next time you can't see the wood for the trees, as the saying goes, literally lift your head and look up. You'll see things you've never noticed before. Changing your perspective can change your life, and it all starts with believing this is possible!

CHAPTER 22

Love and Fear—Choose Love

The most important person to love madly is yourself.

J ohn Lennon's wise quote is one of my favorites: "There are two basic motivating forces: fear and love. When we are afraid, we pull back from life. When we are in love, we open to all that life has to offer with passion, excitement and acceptance. We need to learn to love ourselves first, in all our glory and our imperfections. If we cannot love ourselves, we cannot fully open to our ability to love others or our potential to create. Evolution and all hopes for a better world rest in the fearlessness and open-hearted vision of people who embrace life."

Fear

Our thoughts, words, and actions are either driven by love or fear. Fear is a natural human emotion that is entrenched in our psyche. Fear exists for a reason: to keep us safe. But if we let it, fear can cripple and freeze us in a time and place we don't want to be. When we are afraid, our ego protects us. It convinces us to stay in familiarity. Known discomfort feels safer than uncertainty because we understand exactly what we are dealing with, even if we don't like it. Fear can cause us to stagnate in procrastination and talk us out of making important decisions. Fear caused me to delay booking specialist medical appointments, desperately wanting to avoid the extra stress that these would impose. You may have experienced fear when needing to choose between doctors, fertility options or the timing of treatment, worrying that a wrong decision could be detrimental and need unraveling later. Fear may have subconsciously stopped you from making positive changes to your lifestyle to reduce stress and manage PCOS and infertility better. For example, doing more exercise, changing your diet or beginning to meditate; I know I was guilty of this. The more frequently you inadvertently allow fear to run the show, and repeat these unconscious self-sabotaging patterns of perceived protection, the more deep-rooted they become.

How we respond to fear is therefore imperative. Denying fear or trying to stuff it so far down that we can't feel it is both a waste of energy and counterproductive. Instead, acknowledging fear and beaming a light on it disempowers fear. The pain infertility causes our mind, body and spirit can be torturous, with no guarantee of a baby at the end of it all. This is the greatest fear of all. Making friends with fear is therefore imperative to maintain sanity through the uncertain process. With practice this becomes easier. As American Goodreads author, C. JoyBell C. states so beautifully, "Don't be afraid of your fears. They're not there to scare you. They're there to let you know that something is worth it."[34] If having a baby wasn't so important to you, you wouldn't be afraid of it not working out. So if you can, keep going.

Your fears associated with infertility are understandable, so don't try to push them away. Instead open your heart up and bravely walk toward them. This will lessen their intensity and soften the sharp edges. Paulo Coelho, Brazilian author of *The Alchemist*, says "tell your heart that the fear of suffering is worse than the suffering itself."[35] I learned this through my mindfulness training, and as I reflect on my infertility journey, I know this to be true. I wasted a lot of energy worrying about what may happen and dwelled on things that were out of my control. This didn't change any of the circumstances I faced, and only made me feel worse. For example, my fear of the anticipated suffering caused by going into hospital for a D&C was, on reflection, worse than the experience itself. The good news is that each time you learn this, you're one step closer to being able to change it.

Listening to my guided "Overcoming Fear Meditation" and "Limiting Beliefs Meditation" may help you to understand your fears further. These meditations take you on a journey to face your fears and create space for limiting beliefs and blocks to fully rise to the surface to be healed. They are available to download from my website meditation store.

Once your fears are visible, you can play devil's advocate to them. This is achieved by gently questioning your mind and asking, "Is it real?" for each fear. Doing this helps to bring perspective. You might find that some of your fears, and the possible outcomes that you have imagined, are unlikely to occur. Answering yes or no until every fear has been voiced means many are crossed off the list. Those more emotionally charged and deep-rooted fears, such as never having a baby, can be understood in more detail with transformation coaching and energy healing. This is where incredible healing occurs as you learn to open your heart, ask for help and trust life more.

No matter what PCOS and infertility throw at you, you have the strength to get through it. Back yourself; you have overcome your fears and survived many arduous times in the past. Trust that you can do this again. I believe in you.

Forgiveness

I have learned that forgiveness erases guilt and shame. Forgiveness of self and others is the key that unlocks our heart. But it's not easy.

When I began delving into forgiveness, fear and resistance came up. I was immediately transported back to a time and place I preferred not to be, and in a split second my lacerations were reopened, and the pain, anger and resentment poured from them once more. Reliving those feelings was uncomfortable. *How can I contemplate forgiving those people who have been unsupportive or hurt me with thoughtless words? Why should I let them off the hook? And how can I forgive myself? My body has let me down. It was my fault I was unable to have another child.* These were valid thoughts.

Forgiveness does not excuse behavior or another person's actions. It's not about pretending an incident didn't happen. Forgiveness doesn't alter your past. It is a powerful "inside mind job" requiring unabated strength. But if you graciously accept this, forgiveness can change your future. If you intentionally let go of negative thoughts and emotions toward another person or yourself, forgiveness will free your heart from unnecessary pain and suffering. Forgiveness is freedom, where the reward prevents someone else or yourself from continuing to destroy your life. At last, you can unshackle your heart from the chains that have restricted it so tightly. You can be at peace.

Through hypnotherapy, meditation and writing in my journal, I slowly forgave myself and others. Emotional freedom technique (EFT), or "tapping" as it is also known, is an alternative treatment for physical pain and emotional issues. EFT allowed me to release myself from the past. Letting go of stuff sometimes felt as if I was taking one step forward and two back. But it was worth persisting. I learned how to reevaluate everything, concluding that whether I liked it or not, being human is to make mistakes. We have all made unwise choices and hurt people and ourselves, either unwittingly or otherwise. When we take responsibility, forgiveness can help us heal and grow.

Infertility is an emotional rollercoaster for everyone involved. No one is given a guidebook on how to support themselves or others through this. Perhaps someone has inadvertently hurt you. As much as it wounds us, the disparities that separate us are much smaller than what connects and unites us. Try to meet them halfway, forgive them or say sorry for your part in any misunderstandings. It's never too late to reconnect if you have lost touch. Don't let fear, insecurities or your pride be the reason you didn't. Even if the olive branch is not appreciated or reciprocated, you will have peace in your heart that you tried, rather than suffering through regret.

In 2009, Bronnie Ware wrote a powerful online article called "Regrets of the Dying" about her time as a palliative carer. She went on to share these raw and honest conversations about life and death in her memoir called *The Top Five Regrets of the Dying* which has been read by over a million people. Here are the top five things these patients wished they had done differently[36]:

1. I wish I'd had the courage to live a life true to myself, not the life others expected of me.
2. I wish I hadn't worked so hard.
3. I wish I'd had the courage to express my feelings.
4. I wish I had stayed in touch with my friends.
5. I wish that I had let myself be happier.

If any of these wishes ring true for you, know that it isn't too late to turn this around. Whenever you can, try to enjoy the time you have with family and friends, and make the most of the life you have been given, even if it's not specifically how you would like it to be. I know this is hard. Infertility is full of situations that cannot be controlled, but forgiveness is different. You're fully in charge of this.

Living with regret is not easy, but you can rewrite the ending to this part of your story right now. If you're ready to work on forgiveness, start by downloading my guided "Forgiveness Meditation" from my website meditation store. Or you can listen to this meditation on my YouTube channel called Infertility–Breaking the Silence. You will be surprised by what comes up each time you listen to it.

Self-forgiveness is a key component to living life without regret. I worked on this with energy healers to acknowledge and release the pain and guilt associated with PCOS and infertility that I had subconsciously been holding on to. Self-forgiveness is often the area we try to ignore because it's the hardest, and can be so alien to us. As young children when we make a mistake, we are taught to apologize and forgive others, but never ourselves. So this takes practice. When I forgave myself for my part in my infertility trauma, I felt a huge weight had been lifted from my shoulders. I began to be there for myself, respect and love my body. Forgiveness is love for self. It doesn't get better than that!

The exciting thing about energy is that it has no boundaries, so you can work with a practitioner anywhere in the world. I offer sessions online which enables me to connect with people globally, which I love. Bookings can be made on my website. Forgiveness is life-changing; it sets you free.

Love

Know that love has the potential to heal everything, even your most painful scars. Love opens your heart. The more you connect with your heart, the better you'll feel and the closer you'll be to loving all of you.

As clichéd as it sounds, to love fully, any love story starts with you loving yourself wholeheartedly and unconditionally. Do you love yourself? This is a confronting question. You may have tears in your eyes because you know self-criticism has been a larger part of infertility than self-love and compassion. Don't stop your tears; they will help you release any buried pain you have been ignoring. If you have been focusing on everyone except yourself, it's likely you have forgotten to nourish the most important person in your life and love who you are. Looking in the mirror but with your eyes closed, you might not have seen your own reflection staring back, trying to get your attention. Even if this is the case, it's never too late to begin your journey to self-love.

Self-love quashes fear because you are so strongly connected to your soul, which always guides you in the right direction. Self-love ensures you are not defined by your experiences, and does not let obstacles limit your future. Self-love allows your heart to trust that each piece of your jigsaw puzzle will be revealed at the right time. Regardless of never being able to see the whole picture to your life, you'll reject the notion that taxing periods only have knife-like edges, ugly scenes and dark colors. You'll begin to see that every situation has lighter moments within it too. When you genuinely love yourself, you're less likely to feel as though something is missing. In fact, you will choose to put those same jigsaw pieces back together in precisely the same order. You will recognize that they all make up your beautiful self and that you are already enough. Self-love will help you feel that everything makes perfect sense, despite the heartache of imperfection. Your love for self will beat louder than any niggling doubt that things will not work out in the right way, eventually. Instead, you will have gratitude for the blessings that are also bestowed upon you, even if it's many years from now. Your love for self will make sure of this. When you're faced with the next hurdle in your infertility story, such as miscarriage, self-love will provide you with the courage to get back up quicker. Your love for self will soften your vulnerability and the lingering ache that is caused by trauma, loss and grief.

If you don't yet recognize your full beauty, I hope that this book connects you with your soul and who you truly are. That you feel willing to dive into an exploration of self-love. That you fully invest in yourself, show up and become your most loyal supporter. Keep going until it becomes second nature. This is self-love. Meet fear with love. Choose to love yourself every day, through all the highs and lows of infertility. This will help to fill the hole in your heart. Self-love leads to peace, inner fulfillment, self-acceptance, strength and hope. Loving yourself is the passport to unlocking your future and coping with whatever life throws at you next.

CHAPTER 23

Gratitude Has No Limits

When we focus on gratitude, we are present,
and we attract love, peace, and wisdom.

G ratitude played an essential role in helping me through my inability to conceive, miscarriages, and time in intensive care. No matter how down I got, I also remembered how much I had to be thankful for.

Gratitude Changed My Life

I couldn't have survived my most crushing moments without Giles by my side. My beautiful son Isaac was the guiding light who helped me through all those tough years before we moved to Australia. I have never forgotten the flowers my friend left on my doorstep while I was having my D&C, or the kindness shown by the hospital chaplain. These memories still make me smile. I so appreciated the compassion I received from the Norwegian doctor who came to speak to me and check how I was after her nightshift ended. Each day in hospital I was thankful for the food I ate; it meant I was still alive to enjoy it. Even when I felt broken, gratitude for my family and friends, my supportive boss, and the comfort of my own bed were not lost on me.

After I returned from Norway, I never took my health for granted again. I fell in love with my body and acknowledged all it had done for me by listening to what it needed. When I felt unsupported or ignored, I moved my attention to the other women I had met at a local PCOS group who were also struggling to have a baby and needed kindness. As harsh as those years of infertility were, there was still so much good in my life, with so many things to appreciate. I learned that I shouldn't wait for happiness to start being grateful. Rather, expressing gratitude would naturally bring me more of the joy I desperately craved.

Benefits of Gratitude

Our lives are filled with gifts, but sometimes they get lost in the stress and heartache that infertility brings. Tony Robbins, American coach, speaker, author and philanthropist, highlights that gratitude leads to the following physical health and psychological benefits[37]:

1. Better sleep.
2. Improved heart health.
3. More drive to exercise.
4. Lower blood pressure.
5. Healthier relationships.
6. Decreased negative emotions.
7. Increased empathy.
8. Improved outlook.
9. Higher self-esteem.
10. More inner strength.

It seems counterintuitive to be grateful when facing adversity in life. But expressing gratitude, even for small things, means mental and emotional well-being improves, which aids the management of infertility.

What Gratitude Feels Like

In moments of gratitude, we feel the blessings in our lives and recognize we have all we need. This is different to having all we want. According to American professor and psychologist Robert A. Emmons Ph.D., scientifically speaking, happiness can increase by as much as 25 percent when we have regular grateful thoughts.[38]

Gratitude is powerful because it aligns us with the vibration of love. According to American professor and spiritual teacher Dr. David R. Hawkins, love is the fourth-highest vibrating states of being on his Scale of Consciousness[39]–no wonder it feels so good! Being thankful enables the heart chakra to fully open. So when we practice gratitude, we are also practicing love. An open-heart space allows and attracts more love and abundance, such as deeper relationships, well-being, peace and increased joy into our lives, even during turbulent times such as infertility. Gratitude takes us closer to feeling we are enough.

Expressing Gratitude

I suggest going to the library and seeking out a book on gratitude and infertility. Or you can search for articles and blogs online. The more you understand about gratitude and how it can help you, the more it will resonate with you. You will begin to recognize that moments of deep gratitude keep you present, bring you closer to your true self, and leave an imprint on your heart that material possessions cannot. The next fundamental step is to express gratitude. Doing this each day requires commitment, but it doesn't need to be a time-consuming burden. Here are some simple suggestions:

Gratitude Journals

Gratitude journals are a valuable and easy way to foster the habit of deliberately recognizing and giving thanks for everything that makes life richer. Robert A. Emmons Ph.D. claims that keeping a gratitude diary for twenty-one days can result in better sleep and more energy.[40] I recommend writing down three things you are grateful for either when you first wake up or just before you go to sleep. It only takes five minutes and doesn't have to be anything significant. Simple things, such as being grateful for a hot cup of tea, a good book, a warm shower or a sunny day, remind us of our good fortune. Acknowledging these blessings is powerful and feels good. You might write:

1. I am grateful for… my supportive partner or friend.
2. I am grateful for… my loving pet.
3. I am grateful for… my fire in winter.

Alternatively, answer the following three questions at the end of each day:

1. What did I enjoy the most?
2. Who made me feel good?
3. What made me laugh?

You can also buy an infertility gratitude journal to help you through IVF.

Gratitude Jar

Every day write down or draw three things on small pieces of paper that you are grateful for. Put them in a glass jar. Introduce colored paper and pens to stimulate your creativity. At the end of the week, read them back to yourself or look through the pictures. This will help remind you of all the positivity in your life.

Gratitude Book or Board

Do you relate more to pictures than words? Create a gratitude book or board filled with photos and images from magazines, newspapers or online. Adding color to anything raises your vibration, which is one of the reasons you smile when you see a rainbow. Raising your vibration through color can help you deal better with difficult circumstances. Spend a few minutes every day looking at what you have created.

Meditation

Download my "Gratitude Meditation" from my website meditation store, or there are plenty to choose from on YouTube. Take a breath and see which one you are drawn to. With so many options, you will find something that resonates with you. Notice how you feel after the meditation. Are you lighter, happier?

Gratitude Walk

Go for a walk and pay attention to the stimulation of your senses. Notice and be thankful for the sound of birds chirping in the trees, the smell of fresh coffee as you walk past your favorite café, the sensation you get when someone smiles at you, or the rustle of leaves in the wind.

How Long

Make a concerted effort to practice gratitude for a minimum of twenty-one days. Notice the subtle shift in your energy and those around you. Once you effectively incorporate it into your daily routine, keep going! Remember, the more grateful you are, the more you'll have to be grateful for. It's a win-win!

CHAPTER 24

Grief Following Miscarriage

Grief has no rules or timescales.
Live through it in your own way.

rief is intense sadness or sorrow for what has been lost, and for what will never be. Most of us will grieve at least once in our life. Grief is not something that should be pushed away or resisted, despite how painful it feels. We need to feel our grief to heal and eventually move forward.

When we are grieving, everyone may initially rally around and offer support. But after a certain period, people may be more focused on getting through the uncomfortable moments themselves than being there for us. Others may tiptoe around the subject or avoid it completely in their attempts to not remind us of our loss. Despite being well-intentioned, this behavior still hurts.

When a woman has a miscarriage, she experiences having been physically and mentally prepared for a baby who will never be. Despite the psychological impacts this has on so many couples worldwide, society tends to ignore this taboo subject. Perhaps it's not spoken about because of the body parts involved. My miscarriages exposed me to the silence and social stigma that surrounds infertility, miscarriage, stillbirth, and infant loss. I want to change this. I learned how it feels to grieve deeply and recurrently in relatively short periods of time, behind closed doors.

This hushed form of bereavement showed me how difficult it is to express emotions and grief, despite the loss being very real and painful. Feelings of sadness, loneliness, shame, hopelessness, and deteriorating self-worth were exacerbated further by family and friends not understanding how to support me. They didn't know what to say or what not to say, during some of the toughest years of my life.

Grief is Different for Everyone

We all grieve differently. After my D&C, Giles moved through his grief much quicker than me, coming to a place of acceptance and hope for the future, while I was still angry and depressed. I wish I had understood that there is no right or wrong way to grieve, only our way. If we let it, grief can pull partnerships apart at a time when we need each other the most. I highly recommend grief counseling, either individually or as a couple, so that you can understand how to best support each other. Talking together about the different stages of grief highlighted in figure 2, and acknowledging your unique feelings and thoughts during this heartbreaking time, is also helpful.

Sometimes just having another person outside the relationship who recognizes our pain is enough to help us cope with our grief. The compassion the hospital chaplain showed me, and her acknowledgment that I had lost a baby, helped me heal. Being bombarded with the scientific argument that my baby was only a group of cells that weren't viable never resonated with me. All three of my babies had heartbeats and looked like tiny babies when they died.

Dr. Gunther Von Hagen is a German anatomist who invented plastination, a technique for preserving biological tissue specimens. He showcased his Bodies Exhibition in New York. In 2008, shortly after having my first miscarriage, I visited the fetus section in the exhibition. It was shocking to see how much an embryo looks like a baby, even at eight weeks. It's not surprising, therefore, that miscarriage can be particularly traumatic for women who pass identifiable body parts or who, like me, have already felt their baby moving inside them.

We should not trivialize a woman's experience of losing a baby that has been growing inside her. All life is valuable, regardless of how long that life lived. Someone's importance is not measured by the number of breaths they took. My unborn babies taught me patience, humility and compassion.

Stages of Grief

Elizabeth Kübler-Ross, a Swiss-American psychiatrist, developed a model identifying five stages of grief. Figure 2 is an adaptation of this model, which includes the eight stages I experienced during and after both my miscarriages and IVF cycle. In hindsight, I also grieved when I was diagnosed with PCOS, though didn't recognize this at the time.

This informative guide helps to identify some of the symptoms of grief and what stage you or a loved one could be going through. It is important to remember, however, that we do not "get over" grief by a specific time, and there's individual variation. The stages, therefore, need to be loosely interpreted. Grief is not an activity that enables us to progress onto the next stage once we have ticked off each aspect in the previous box. The stages can be hit simultaneously. We can also move backward and forward through the stages more than once, and they can take place out of order. Understanding this means we can focus on the present, which is the best place to heal, and how to support ourselves and others through grief.

Stage of Grief	Symptom of Grief
Shock	Numbed disbelief Initial paralysis
Denial	Avoidance of pain and confusion Fear Sadness
Anger	Frustration gives way to anger Blame others for death, or mistakes that lead to death Irritation or anxiety
Bargaining	Reach out to others/repeatedly tell story Struggle to find meaning Question: "Why me?" Bargain: "I'll exercise more if you bring my baby back."
Depression	Overwhelm, hopelessness, hostility, flight Realization that death is certain Reflect on memories Shut others out/isolate self Cry a lot or become silent Emotional reactions (panic, anxiety, nightmares, fear)

Guilt	Remorse over things did/didn't do while pregnant
Acceptance	Physical symptoms subside (disturbed sleep patterns, low energy, poor appetite, pain) Depression lifts a little See light at the end of the tunnel Find the way forward and move on Reconstruct self and adjust to life without baby
Hope	Think about lost baby without pain Anticipate good times to come Find joy in life

Figure 2: Eight Stages of Grief Following Miscarriage

*Adaptation of Elizabeth Kübler-Ross's Five Stages of Grief Cycle

Communicating with and Supporting Someone who is Grieving

Until we have walked a mile in their shoes, we don't understand the trials people face and the pain they bear. I inadvertently said insensitive things I regret before I experienced infertility, miscarriage and grief.

Ill-considered words such as the ones highlighted in figure 3 bruise us. I still remember the most upsetting ones voiced to me when I was unable to conceive, and recovering from my miscarriages and IVF cycle. By raising awareness of what not to say and do, together we can be more mindful of our words and actions during these sensitive times.

We can't take away each other's pain, but there are numerous ways to communicate with and support someone who is experiencing grief. Suggested words and gestures that lighten stress and bring real comfort are highlighted in figure 4. If you find it difficult to articulate your feelings and explain how someone could help ease your suffering, sharing this chapter with your family and friends may be beneficial.

Miscarriage and Grief—20 Things Not to Say and Do	
"How are you?"	When we say this we mean well. The response, however, will likely be "fine" or "okay" instead of expressing true feelings.

"You're coping with this better than I thought you would." or **"You seem to be doing okay."**	We shouldn't make assumptions about how someone is feeling. They may be putting on a brave face and are actually struggling privately. If someone senses your relief that they are seemingly doing okay, it may be harder for them to be honest and admit they're not.
"Going out will make you feel better."	It's normal to be depressed and not feel like going out. Even though a change of scenery is good for the mind, body and spirit, they may not be ready to distract themselves from their grief. It's best not to put this pressure on them.
"Please let me know if there is anything I can do for you."	This puts responsibility and pressure on someone who is grieving to reach out for help when they're feeling vulnerable. They may not know what they need or be able to muster the courage to ask for help. As well-intentioned as your words are, don't wait to be asked, act.
"I know how you feel."	None of us ever knows what someone else is feeling, even if we have been through a similar experience. Each miscarriage or loss is unique and personal.
"Stay positive/strong." or **"Don't cry."**	These words come from a compassionate place but are inadvertently dismissing or shutting down someone else's feelings and true emotions. Doing this when they are potentially at their most vulnerable is particularly insensitive. Sadness is a normal reaction that needs to be expressed, and being able to do so is a sign of strength, not weakness. Try listening more and saying less.
"Miscarriage is common."	It's true that miscarriage is common. But saying this minimizes grief and implies that because it's frequent, losing a pregnancy matters less.
"Aren't you over your miscarriage yet?" or **"It's time to move on."**	It's not for us to judge when someone should have healed from their miscarriage. Recovery and grief have no timescales; everyone grieves at their own speed. Instead we need to offer reassurance that grief is natural.

"It was a group of cells, not a baby." or **"At least it wasn't actually a baby."**	Even though a doctor may perceive the loss as a group of cells, to that family they have lost their baby. These words hurt.
"At least you weren't further along."	Regardless of how far along someone was in their pregnancy, the end result is still the same: no baby. While grieving, people are not able to see a bright side of their physical and emotional trauma.
"There was obviously something wrong with the baby." or **"It's for the best."**	Hearing that someone thinks losing an unborn baby is best for them is really hard to process. Even if there could have been a medical explanation, these statements are dismissive and provide no comfort.
"Everything happens for a reason." or **"Your baby came here for a reason."**	Suggesting there's a reason behind their baby's death doesn't make the loss any easier to endure. These words are not the perceived silver lining anyone needs to hear, particularly when grief is raw. It is therefore advisable to avoid phrases like these.
"Your baby is in a better place." or **"Your baby wasn't part of God's plan."**	Even if a baby was suffering in the womb or shortly after birth, these words may be painful to hear. Faith-based ideas should be avoided. We cannot know what someone's belief system is or how comments like these will impact them. Regardless of where a baby has gone to, they are not with their parents and that's what makes loss so hard.
"It wasn't your baby's time." or **"It was their time to go."**	At a time when miscarriage may feel senseless, or when someone is grieving, no death can be justified.
"At least you know you can get pregnant."	Some women don't ever fall pregnant which is devastating. Miscarriage, however, also leads to the same outcome: no baby. We don't know how long it took someone to conceive and what they have already been through (appointments, tests, hormones, IVF treatments and financial stress) to get to the pregnancy they lost. The reason for a miscarriage may never be identified, falling pregnant again may not be easy, and future miscarriages may be feared.

"Just relax."	For anyone battling with infertility, "just relax" is the most common–and worst–unsolicited advice to receive. This is dismissive and minimizes a woman's feelings.
"You can always have another baby." or "I'm sure you'll have another baby." or "When you have another baby, you won't be able to imagine life with a different one."	These words minimalize the pregnancy that has just been lost. I felt like screaming, "I wanted that baby." None of my miscarried babies were replaceable. Even though I wouldn't have my two divine daughters if I hadn't lost my three babies, I have never forgotten them. Miscarriage reminds us that nothing is certain, we have little control, and life is not always fair and this can be confronting. "I'm sure you will have another baby" is also an empty promise. Having another baby is not guaranteed for many couples who have already tried for years to conceive. Fertility treatment is expensive and may be out of reach. These words dismiss valid concerns.
"You can adopt. There are lots of children who need homes."	The desire to have a biological child is very real. While these options may have been or may need to be considered, this discussion usually means many doors have been shut on the road to parenthood, hope has been lost and much heartache endured. This is, therefore, always a subject to tread very carefully around.
Nothing at all.	It shocked, puzzled and hurt me how many people remained silent, never reached out and avoided the subject altogether. When I was most vulnerable, it felt like some people didn't care. On reflection, I know this was probably because they were uncomfortable or didn't know what to say. However, I would have preferred someone to try, even if they didn't get it quite right, rather than ignore this painful subject altogether.
Not seeking permission before discussing publicly or posting on social media.	Someone may want to share their loss in their own way and at the right time for them. Because there's little control in the grieving process, it's best not to take this aspect away from them as well.

Figure 3: Miscarriage and Grief—20 Things Not to Say and Do

Miscarriage and Grief—20 Things to Say and Do	
"I'm sorry for your and your partner's loss. I'm here for you both." or **"I wish I had the right words. I care and am here for you."**	These simple statements can be so appreciated by a couple who are grieving. Partners often get forgotten, so these words show you care about them both. Not everyone is good with their words, but feeling supported is invaluable. We can show we care through eye contact, gestures, being attentive, and listening.
"You're in my thoughts." or **"I love you."**	Even though no one can fix it, knowing that someone is thinking of them or loves them means the world. Love heals.
"I don't know how you are feeling. I am here to help in any way I can."	This communicates concern but is not assuming you understand how they feel or what's best for them.
"Grief is natural; it takes time." or **"It's okay to not be feeling great."**	These words validate feelings. It's comforting to be reassured that there's nothing wrong with them, that grief takes time and each moment without their baby is difficult.
"You're suffering; I'm so sorry." or **"This must be really difficult for you right now."** or **"I know it's hard to be strong at the moment."**	Acknowledging someone's pain shows compassion and gives them chance to grieve without feeling judged. Chances are they're already exhausted from dealing with countless infertility hurdles, and now loss. So giving them permission to not be strong all the time is freeing.
"I know others who've had a miscarriage and how much grief they felt. I'm aware this is difficult for you."	Conveying another person's experience, or your own, without comparing, provides hope that they'll be able to move on when they're ready. Importantly though, it doesn't dismiss how hard the struggle currently is.
"This was not your fault." or **"Nothing you have or haven't done could have changed the outcome."**	It's common for women who have suffered a miscarriage to question themselves, feel guilty and wonder what they did wrong. Even though logically they know miscarriage is never their fault, it's comforting to hear this from those they respect and trust.
"There was no good reason for your baby to be taken from you."	Expressing this can help someone who is grieving feel validated and heard.

"You must really miss being pregnant; I'm sorry."	It takes time to adjust physically and mentally to no longer being pregnant. Acknowledging this, rather than brushing it aside, validates their loss.
"Try to be kind to yourself."	Self-care is often not prioritized. Yet showing kindness to the most eminent person in their life is vital. Reminding someone to be kind to themselves when they are suffering can help the healing process. Simple things like putting moisturizer on, sitting under a tree, or curling up on the sofa for an afternoon nap are all nurturing.
"Can I give you a hug?"	Asking permission to hug someone or sitting quietly with a box of tissues and holding space for them can be all that is needed. Reminding them that you are there for them and it's okay to cry is reassuring.
"At times like this we all need help." or **"You're not alone. I will help you through this tough time."**	Validating that you understand they're not going to feel 100 percent helps to remove the pressure to snap out of it and move on. These simple words can mean so much to someone when they are grieving. Encouraging them to express their pain and stress will help healing to occur.
"I am usually up early or late, so please feel comfortable phoning or texting for a chat if you ever need anything."	Grief can play havoc with sleeping patterns. This adds to feelings of loneliness during the middle of the night. Knowing that someone may be awake at odd hours, even just to answer a few text messages, can provide huge comfort.
"Would you like to go to the event/activity together?"	Suggesting going to an event together is an enormous emotional support. Walking into a room alone can be confronting, and even harder when someone is grieving.
"I'll come round for a cup of coffee."	Being with someone when they are grieving brings comfort. A book, cake, or a care package with tea, tissues and a heartfelt card can be thoughtful presents. Sometimes it's easier to write emotions down than vocalize them, so a special notebook and pen might be appreciated. Grief doesn't end after a few weeks or months, so regular visits may be welcomed.

"I'll pick up groceries each week." or **"I'll drop round dinner every Monday night."** or **"I'll come by and do the laundry."**	Performing household chores can relieve daily burdens. It's easier for someone to accept specific help because the person offering is willing and capable. It also takes pressure off them having to come up with ideas when their world has been turned upside down.
"If you'd like to honor your baby, I'd be happy to help you organize this or come along for support."	My baby's funeral service helped to provide closure. Holding a private ceremony with candles and saying special words, or planting a tree in the back garden, can be very healing and honor the life that has been lost.
Express your condolences privately. "I'm sorry, I love you and I'm here for you."	We have forgotten the artform of direct communication. Instead of posting condolences on social media, phone, leave a message, or send a card or private message to show you care. "I'm sorry, I love you and I'm here for you" is a powerful message.
Read miscarriage, grief and bereavement literature.	This will help you feel more comfortable supporting someone who is grieving.
Recognize that grandparents can hurt twice.	Hurting twice as a grandparent is common. Once for their hurting child, and once for the grandchild they have lost. Memories of their past pregnancy losses may resurface. Talking about feelings facilitates grieving and healing.

Figure 4: Miscarriage and Grief—20 Things to Say and Do

We are designed to be part of a community and be involved in one another's lives, both in the good times and the bad. Grief is the worst pain someone can endure; we are not meant to handle this alone. It's our role to lift each other up and reach out when we see someone struggling with the burden of grief.

Miscarriage and stillbirth are silent forms of bereavement. We all play a part in shining a light on this, so that those contending with infertility no longer grieve alone. Listening, being compassionate and respecting boundaries is a great place to start. Allowing loved ones to grieve on their own terms and in their own timescales is important. An apology for saying the wrong thing usually helps to lessen any hurt. We are all doing our best.

And no matter whether we are dealing with miscarriage, grieving or supporting someone else who is grieving, we should accept that we are in charge of how we respond (not react) to other people and what life throws at us. Breathing and taking a metaphorical step back from the situation, just for a moment, helps to stop misunderstandings from escalating; there is enough to contend with already.

When we question if we can let it go and whether our energy is better focused elsewhere, chances are the answer is yes. Responding brings calm, softness and space to communication and our interactions with others. This reduces stress which is essential for the infertility journey.

CHAPTER 25

Growing Through the Pain

*We must be there for ourselves, throughout all the mess
and heartache. We need to be our best friend
when no one else knows how.*

Infertility, just like life, is full of uncertainty and change. Neither is easy to
deal with. Going through fertility treatment, such as IVF, is a heavy reminder
about how unpredictable life is and how little control we have.

Dealing with Uncertainty and Change

We know a positive mindset is important to increase the chances of falling pregnant. Yet we fear having our hopes too high during the two-week wait in case the
treatment isn't successful and we end up back where we started. Scheduling in
lots of rest and distracting our wandering minds with fun times can reduce the
pressure and expectation we inadvertently place on ourselves. Trying not to be
influenced by others and really listening to what we specifically need is valuable.
Whether we take time off work, keep a regular routine, or go on holiday, it's an
ideal opportunity to practice self-care.

During my infertility journey, I learned that nobody else could heal me.
Inside me lay the strength I needed to move forward after each setback so I could

lessen my suffering. Ironically, knowing this gave me back my power and some control. The only way to change how I felt was to be present with my pain. This was uncomfortable, but necessary.

This new way of being is also available to you. If there's no positive pregnancy test, be kind to yourself and try to remember that nothing lasts forever. This pain that you are feeling right now will change and eventually soften. Keep holding on to hope that your time will come.

Guilt, Failure, and Shame

Guilt, failure, and shame are complex emotions experienced during infertility. Throughout my quest to have a second child, I mentally beat myself up about the following:

1. My body not working properly/failing myself and others.
2. Not being able to give Giles a second child.
3. Isaac being lonely and growing up without a sibling.
4. Feeling guilty about being angry with the medical professionals when they made mistakes or ignored me (deep down I knew they were doing their best).
5. Being frustrated that I had no control over anything.
6. Feeling impatient.
7. Voicing my pain. I knew others were waiting to have their first child, whereas I already had one which led to feelings of guilt.
8. Not loving myself through infertility.
9. Being jealous when other people fell pregnant.
10. Not being able to feel more positive and becoming a negative person.

Adding guilt as a second emotion on top of everything else I was feeling only exacerbated the underlying shame. This felt particularly unpleasant; shame is the lowest vibration emotion. At the time I didn't understand that this was what I was doing, and I didn't have the tools to know how to stop. If you are experiencing any of these feelings, I encourage you to talk about them. Shining a light on shame softens it and takes away its power. Meditation and going out into nature more often quietens the critical thoughts. Balance your mind with affirmations, and spend time with your tribe and those you trust. Anyone who can help pick you back up when you feel as though the world is against you is worth spending your time with.

NICU and Breastfeeding

Before I had Isaac, I didn't know that my PCOS meant I was at an increased risk of giving birth prematurely. I blamed my body, despite having no control over this, because I didn't know what else to believe. Isaac's prematurity and breastfeeding issues were not my fault, but unfortunately it wasn't the message I heard. I felt so much guilt and grief. I felt like a failure.

My heart broke each time I left the hospital without Isaac. I felt guilty for leaving him lying alone in a plastic box at night instead of in my arms. I grieved for the precious moments we missed out on shortly after Isaac's birth and while he was in hospital. I felt guilty, on top of feeling grief, because even though I was grateful that my beautiful baby was okay, this wasn't enough to erase the grief that clung to my heavy heart. When I learned that bottle-feeding Isaac would have brought him home sooner from hospital, guilt set in that I didn't ask more questions. Hindsight is a wonderful thing. But when I took the step of bottle-feeding him, I felt guilty and like a failure for not breastfeeding him. When Isaac had developmental delays and was diagnosed with dyspraxia at five years old, I felt the old feelings of failure, guilt, shame and grief sporadically resurface for years. I still have moments where I feel sadness about the things Isaac is still unable to do, and the struggles he has endured.

If I had understood the extra stress Isaac's prematurity caused my mind, body and spirit, and that I was grieving, I would have been much more empathetic toward myself. Time does heal once emotions have been processed. Today I have forgiven myself, and can see the positive in each situation that we have overcome, but it was a tough ride getting to this point.

If you are blessed with a baby and go through any of these challenges, I am here to remind you that it is not your fault. Be gentle with yourself along the way. Allow yourself to feel what you feel without judgment. If your baby ends up in NICU, celebrate each small milestone, knowing you are a step closer to taking your baby home. Try to be patient while you wait, but don't rebuke yourself when you're not. Do nice things for yourself to aid your recovery. Take warm baths, get plenty of rest, eat nutritious food and breathe in fresh air. Soon your baby will be in your arms, where they belong.

Trust Your Instinct

Throughout this book I have spoken about allowing self-doubt to prohibit my ability to speak up for myself, even when I knew something wasn't quite right. I kept quiet for too long before my PCOS diagnosis, while in early labor with Isaac, and when I was in hospital in Norway. Not wanting to cause a fuss and worrying that I was a fraud did me no favors.

What I have learned since is that you will be guided in the right direction when you connect deeply with self, search for the answers inside you, and trust your intuition, even when others doubt you. I encourage you to listen to your body because you understand it better than anybody else. Keep asking doctors questions, and seek second opinions when needed. Never be afraid to speak your truth. If something doesn't feel right, it probably isn't. You may not want to offend your specialist, but your well-being is more important than any temporary embarrassment you or they may feel. Always attend each medical appointment with your list of questions written down. It can be hard to remember everything you wanted to ask when emotions are running high. Understanding what tests are available, the side effects of any medications you are instructed to take, the likelihood of success, alternative options, timescales and next steps will help you feel more empowered that you are making the right choices, and alleviate some of the stress endured.

Infertility and Friendship

Infertility can put a great strain on friendships; I know you may have already experienced this. I wrongly assumed that because I had supported friends through their miscarriages that they would be there for me. Unfortunately, the very topic that had previously united and bonded us was no longer discussed once their second children were born.

At the time, I felt frustrated and abandoned, but was unable to articulate this. In hindsight I realize that placing expectations on others only leads to hurt.

In an ideal world, we would have all spoken about this subject before any of us conceived again, foreseeing that it could be difficult on each side. I encourage you to do this. I appreciated that the organizer of my PCOS support group sought agreement from members on how she could best communicate that someone had fallen pregnant. It was her diplomacy that kept the group intact. Connecting with these women earlier in my journey would have taken the pressure off my existing friendships. This may be worth considering for yourself.

Today I can also look at this situation slightly differently. I understand that friends come and go, which is a necessary part of life. With the lapsing of one friendship, space was made for new friendships where I could grow with women I was better energetically aligned with for the next chapter. Despite it being painful, I encourage you to bring this new perspective to the situation, if only to maintain your sanity! Be your own best friend and love yourself more fiercely throughout your heartache. When you don't receive the love and support you desire from others, go inwards and be there for yourself unconditionally.

CHAPTER 26

Your Future without a Baby

*Accepting that life is different to the one
we dreamed about takes great courage.*

I can't imagine how it feels to endure the painful infertility rollercoaster without being able to hold a baby in your arms at the end of it all. Whether doctors have told you fertility treatment options have been exhausted, or you have decided to stop trying for physical, mental, emotional or financial reasons, my heart goes out to you. I am so sorry.

I understand it may not be possible for you to articulate the heartbreak and isolation you feel, or know how to face a life that looks nothing like the one you had planned. Please nurture yourself through the pain and uncertainty. Be vulnerable, reach out to others and ask for help. When you are ready, join support groups and read articles written by those who do understand the journey. Connect with other women and couples who have walked this road before you. Their stories will give you strength and inspiration to move forward. We all need connection, and it is this support from others that will guide you through these dark times to a place of acceptance.

Never stop loving yourself. Please know this chapter in your life does not define you. With or without a baby, you are always enough. I am sending you much love, healing and courage.

CHAPTER 27

Toolbox and Resources

Together we can overcome our pain and rise once again.

Burying, resisting or denying our grief does not make this pain disappear; we just carry it with us for longer. Tightly holding on to what we have been through and making it our story means we are in danger of remaining stuck, and inadvertently allowing our past trauma to define us and our future.

It's important to allow ourselves space and time to open up to feeling the emotions and pain without judgment. We can then release everything from our bodies and move forward. This chapter includes various tools and resources to support you through your trauma, so that you can process your emotions and begin to heal.

Rituals and Private Ceremonies After Loss

Coming to terms with any loss is not easy. A ritual brings a glimmer of light into the surrounding dark fog. Honoring the memory of your baby through a private ceremony can be healing. My baby's funeral service helped to provide closure; I have such gratitude for this.

Three Rituals for Miscarriages

1. Hold a ceremony or memorial service in a special place or at home. You may wish to do this alone, with your partner, or invite family and close friends. Poems or prayers such as the ones included in Part One of this book could be shared. Or you may prefer to write your own poem or a letter to your baby. Lighting candles and expressing the dreams you had for your baby, or how you envisioned your future together, can be cathartic. Letting-go rituals, such as blowing bubbles or throwing petals into the ocean, begin the healing process.

2. Plant a rose bush or fruit tree so that life continues. As each season passes you will have a unique reminder of their love. This growing plant or tree also gives you a physical space to grieve in, which may bring you comfort.

3. Paint a picture, create a paper or digital collage, make an object out of clay, or write and record some special music. Being creative helps you connect with your heart. Color heals, so choose tones and textures that you are naturally drawn to.

Infertility Coaching and Energy Healing

I offer individual and couples infertility coaching and energy healing. Our sessions are focused on balancing the mind, body and spirit so you are in the best place possible to welcome a baby into the world. Go to my website for more information.

Grief Meditation

If you have suffered a miscarriage or had a stillborn baby, you know only too well the grief that follows loss. Grief can be all-consuming, particularly after any form of trauma. Nurture yourself. If you are feeling alone, misunderstood and overwhelmed by grief, my guided "Grief Meditation" may help you to release your tears and heal. This meditation can be downloaded at my website meditation store.

Olivia Fox's Song about Miscarriage

I highly recommend following the American band, Oliva Fox. Their moving song, "Elevator Doors," was written about the day Lauren Flynn, the lead singer-songwriter, discovered she was miscarrying her baby. The lyrics about the only sound in the ultrasound room being silence, and questioning why her baby came if they weren't going to stay, resonated with me so deeply that I reached out to her for a chat. Our conversation about miscarriage, grief and the silence surrounding these subjects can be listened to on my website[41] or YouTube channel.[42] Please share "Elevator Doors" and our discussion with anyone who has faced miscarriage and would benefit from hearing that they are not alone. You can connect with Oliva Fox through their website and social media platforms.[43]

The "Heartache to Hope" Podcast

The "Heartache to Hope" podcast is a space where Anita Thompson and her guests get real about infertility, IVF, miscarriage, and so much more. Anita shares her personal heartbreaking story to help others feel less alone. She also interviews ordinary women who have become extraordinary through their journeys. Anita's intention is to support people through their heartache and find their hope, whatever that looks like. My episode of this podcast and many others are available to listen to at Apple Podcasts[44] or on all the main podcast platforms. You can connect with Anita via her website[45] and social media.[46]

Infertility Support for Men

Men often get forgotten about on the path to parenthood and there isn't as much support available for them. "IVF Dad" is a podcast hosted by Chris Lawson which I highly recommend encouraging male partners to listen to. This podcast candidly shares the "heartache, pain, wacky diets, excitement, hope, determination and loss of faith"[47] that Chris and his wife, Patricia, went through. After five years of trying for a baby, a lot of needles, countless rounds of IVF, eighteen embryos and a rollercoaster ride through infertility treatment, their daughter Rosie was born in January 2020. This IVF success story is available to listen to on the "IVF Dad" website[48] and all the usual podcast platforms.

Infertility Support for the LGBTQIA+ Community

I recommend anyone who is struggling with infertility within the LGBTQIA+ community to seek support from specialists such as Rainbow Infertility via their website.[49] They are the first dedicated fertility and IVF service provider in Australia to cater exclusively for the LGBTQIA+ community. They offer counseling and help people to achieve their dream of becoming a parent. I encourage you to search for a similar local organization.

Three Little Birds Perinatal is based in the USA. They offer pregnancy and infant loss support to families at no cost. You can read more about the support they offer to the LGBTQIA+ community on their website.[50]

There are also LGBTQIA+ support groups within Facebook and on other social media platforms for those going through infertility or supporting their partner through it.

SANDS Worldwide Association

SANDS is an independent organization that provides support for miscarriage, stillbirth and newborn death. This group is based in the UK, but there are also other groups around the world. You can connect with them at their UK website[51] and Australian website.[52] I encourage you to search for your own local organizations and associations; you are not alone.

The Pink Elephants Support Network

Based in Australia, this network supports people through miscarriage and early pregnancy loss. They offer online group support programs and emotional support resources. You can find them via their website.[53]

World Infertility Awareness Month

World Infertility Awareness Month is celebrated every June across the globe to increase awareness regarding infertility issues faced by couples. This includes problems related to female as well as male fertility. Connect with local organizations to find out what events are taking place near you.

National Infertility Awareness Week (NIAW)

NIAW is a movement founded in 1989 by RESOLVE: The National Infertility Association. Its mission is to empower people to change the conversation around infertility. Their website[54] contains the specific dates in April that this takes place each year.

Baby Loss Awareness Week (Miscarriage, Stillbirth, SIDS, and Newborn Death)

Baby Loss Awareness Week runs annually from the 9th to the 15th of October. This ends on Pregnancy and Infant Loss Remembrance Day, on the 15th of October, with the Global Wave of Light. People from around the world are invited to light a candle at 7:00 p.m. local time in memory of all the babies who lit up our lives for only a short time. More support and information is available on their website.[55]

Alternative Therapies

Nature has been the best healing therapy for me. I also recommend trying alternative therapies to help balance emotions and manage the physical side effects of drugs. Reflexology, hypnotherapy, reiki, energy healing, kinesiology and emotional freedom technique (EFT) have benefited me over the years. I have heard positive reviews about acupuncture but was never brave enough to subject myself to more needles!

Final Words

When your mind tries to convince you that hope has been lost, listen to your heart. Your heart will encourage you to look for solutions and keep moving forward. Hope will help you to face your challenges. All pain is temporary and better times lay ahead. Your strength comes from within. No matter what happens, trust yourself and know that you will be okay. You are loved. You are love.

Keep Growing and Discovering

Thank you for sharing this book with me and beginning to reflect on your life. I would love for us to continue working together.

1:1 Coaching

Infertility coaching is available either individually, as a couple, or a combination of both these options at www.sarahwilloughby.com.au/infertilitycoaching. To embark on a deeper journey of healing and self-discovery, book one-on-one coaching sessions at www.sarahwilloughby.com.au/transformationcoaching.

Reiki

To experience this natural energy-balancing method of Japanese healing in person, or to receive a distant healing, go to www.sarahwilloughby.com.au/reiki.

Meditations

If you enjoyed the meditations mentioned in this book, download a range of other meditations at www.sarahwilloughby.com.au/meditation-store.

Subscribe to My List

Receive a free guided "Breathing Meditation," guidance and special offers by subscribing to my newsletter at www.sarahwilloughby.com.au.

Free Videos and Meditations

Subscribe to my YouTube channel: Infertility–Breaking the Silence www.youtube.com/channel/UCj7B9AAPLyGDci2Y6tvoMVw.

Stay in Touch

Website: www.sarahwilloughby.com.au.

LinkedIn: sarahwilloughby-2019 www.linkedin.com/in/sarah-willoughby-2019.

Facebook page and Infertility Saved My Life group: @SarahWilloughbyAustralia. www.facebook.com/SarahWilloughbyAustralia.

Instagram: @sarahwilloughbyaustralia www.instagram.com/sarahwilloughbyaustralia.

YouTube: Infertility–Breaking the Silence www.youtube.com/channel/UCj7B9AAPLyGDci2Y6tvoMVw.

Connect

To connect with the people mentioned in this book, head over to my website www.sarahwilloughby.com.au/infertilitysavedmylife.

Acknowledgments

I nfertility *Saved My Life: Healing PCOS from the Inside Out* began in 2017. Somehow in its own time, and at the right time, this story eventually came together. I am now proud to release this with love to the world.

I would like to express my gratitude to everyone who contributed in some way to this book coming to fruition.

First and foremost, thank you to my beautiful family. Isaac, Madison, Grace and Giles: you are such a blessing in my life. Thank you for encouraging me to share my story, even when the consequence was time apart. Your unconditional love and support mean everything to me and I could not have accomplished this without you.

To all the medical professionals involved in my care over so many years, you are the reason I have three amazing children. Thank you.

I would like to thank David Hancock and the team at Morgan James Publishing for believing in my story. Thank you to all those talented individuals who were instrumental in the creation of this book, especially Jim Howard, Gayle West and Heidi Nickerson.

To my wonderful editors, Samantha Sainsbury, Ann Bolch, Frances Madigan, and Cortney Donelson. Thank you for encouraging me and helping to bring my story alive. I have learned so much from working with all of you. Your patience, compassion, and love for writing are undeniable.

And finally, my heart is deeply grateful to you. Thank you for being called to pick up this book and share it with others. May you follow your heart, go on a journey to self-love, heal past hurts and live the life you are so deserving of.

With love, Sarah x

About the Author

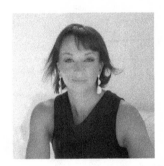

S arah Willoughby is an infertility coach, transformation coach, speaker, reiki practitioner and energy healer. She is also a co-author for the international best seller Business, *Life and the Universe, Volume Three*.

Passionate about guiding people through a journey to self-love, Sarah empowers people to heal, achieve more and transform their lives. Regularly appearing on global podcasts, interviews and speaking panels, Sarah shares her story and messages of hope. She believes that the answer to every problem we face lies inside ourselves; we just need to connect and tune in. As a result of her work, Sarah has an expanding worldwide social media following on LinkedIn, Facebook, Instagram and YouTube.

Prior to following her spiritual path, Sarah forged a successful ten-year career in human resources, working at world-renowned organizations. During this time, meditation and mindfulness became increasingly important as she coped with secondary infertility. In 2009, Sarah's admission into ICU after a disastrous IVF cycle tremendously changed her perspective on life. Seven months later, she emigrated to Australia from the UK with her family, left the corporate world, fell pregnant naturally and began a new life coaching healing, writing and speaking. Sarah loves supporting people to understand the connection between their mind, body and spirit, and how this impacts their journey to parenthood.

Sarah is blessed to live by the beach near Melbourne. Here she can be found enthusiastically writing her way around cafés and spending time in nature with her three incredible children.

Fact Sheet about
Polycystic Ovary Syndrome (PCOS)

What is Polycystic Ovary Syndrome (PCOS)?

Polycystic Ovary Syndrome (PCOS), is a complex hormonal condition that can affect reproduction, metabolism, and emotional health and well-being. "Polycystic" literally means "many cysts"[56] but this name is misleading. The dark areas seen on an ultrasound are follicles or underdeveloped eggs within the ovaries, not cysts. A woman with PCOS has higher levels of insulin and androgens which means her ovaries work differently. Mature eggs may not be released from the ovary every month (ovulation), resulting in irregular menstrual cycles.

How Common is PCOS?

According to the U.S. Department of Health and Human Services, "PCOS is a health problem that affects one in ten women of childbearing age."[57] In the UK, one in five women is affected by PCOS.[58] Within Australia, up to one in eight women of reproductive age is impacted.[59]

How is PCOS Diagnosed?

Jean Hailes for Women's Health states that two out of the following three characteristics must be present for a diagnosis to be confirmed:

1. Menstrual problems (irregular or absent periods).
2. Symptoms (scalp hair loss, increased facial and/or body hair growth, acne, or higher levels of androgen (male type) hormones confirmed by a blood test).
3. Polycystic ovaries (twenty or more follicles on either ovary) found by ultrasound.[60]

PCOS continues to be challenging for women and their health professionals and remains poorly understood, which leads to delays in diagnosis, inconsistent treatment and lack of support.[61] Unfortunately, even though there are vast numbers of women all around the world dealing with PCOS, it appears they are still not receiving the support and care they desperately need. Not only are women suffering, but those closest to them are also impacted.

What Causes PCOS?

Increased levels of the male hormones known as androgens (including testosterone) are often found in women with PCOS, as well as the hormone insulin. Insulin resistance is thought to be the main problem driving this syndrome, but the cause has not been determined. In some women, there is a genetic link. PCOS runs in the family. For others, the condition only occurs when they are overweight. Despite polycystic ovaries (PCO) being seen by ultrasound in up to a third of women, they do not all have PCOS.

PCOS Symptoms[62]

Women who have PCOS may experience all or some of the following symptoms:

1. Irregular menstrual cycles. Bleeding may vary in frequency due to less frequent ovulation (production of an egg).
2. No menstrual period, sometimes for many years.
3. Irregular spotting.
4. Reduced fertility (difficulty in becoming pregnant)–related to infrequent ovulation or absent ovulation.
5. Greater risk of recurrent miscarriage.

6. Anxiety and depression.

7. Emotional distress, mood swings and low self-esteem.

8. Body-image challenges and increased risk of eating disorders.

9. Increased risk of weight gain and obesity.

10. Excess body and facial hair.

11. Scalp hair loss in the central part of the scalp.

12. Acne or pimples.

13. Dark patches of skin.

14. Increased heart disease risk factors including higher cholesterol levels.

15. Higher risk of adult-onset prediabetes or type 2 diabetes.

16. Higher risk of diabetes in pregnancy.

17. Sleep apnea.

18. Chronic fatigue.

19. Dizziness and an increased tendency to faint.

20. Breast, abdominal and pelvic pain.

21. Aching joints.

*Please note: you do not need to have all these symptoms to have PCOS.

Treatment for PCOS

There is no cure for PCOS. It is a lifelong condition, but symptoms can be managed. Throughout the past thirty-odd years of living with PCOS, both my symptoms and their management have changed. If you are seeking a reference book discussing PCOS or infertility from a medical perspective, including the signs, symptoms and support services available, I recommend reading *PCOS* by Colette Harris with Dr. Adam Carey. This book proved to be invaluable when I was first diagnosed and still sits on my bookshelf.

It's vital to obtain the relevant advice that's needed and warranted for your individual condition. This will depend on your symptoms, age and life phase. Treatment for PCOS includes a healthy lifestyle, weight loss if overweight, and targeted therapy such as hormones and medication.[63] In Part Two, I share what techniques and therapies specifically worked for me, and how I improved my relationship with PCOS, so that you can do the same.

Endnotes

1   Miya Yamamoto, MD, et al.. "Risk of Preterm Delivery in Non-Diabetic Women with Polycystic Ovarian Syndrome." National Center for Biotechnology Information. 19 Jan 2012, accessed 29 Feb 2022, http://www.ncbi.nlm.nih.gov/pmc/articles/PMC3570271.

2   The Women's Royal Hospital website. "Miscarriage." Accessed 28 Feb 2022, https://www.thewomens.org.au/health-information/pregnancy-and-birth/pregnancy-problems/early-pregnancy-problems/miscarriage.

3   The Women's Royal Hospital. "Miscarriage."

4   Carla Cain Walther. "What Every Woman Needs to Know about a Silent or Missed Miscarriage." Sofeminine Blog post, 16 Oct 2014, accessed 28 Feb 2022, https://www.sofeminine.co.uk/conception/missed-miscarriage-silent-miscarriage-mmc-lost-baby-s1071286.html.

5   The Women's Royal Hospital. "Miscarriage."

6   Wikipedia. "Breathworks." Accessed 28 Feb 2022, https://en.wikipedia.org/wiki/Breathworks.

7   IVF1 website. "Frozen Embryo Transfer Success." Accessed 28 Feb 2022, https://www.ivf1.com/frozen-embryo-transfer-success.

8   Material from Joe Dispenza. Unlimited website, https://drjoedispenza.com.

9   Joe Dispenza. Hay House World Summit Interview, 2016.

10 Chopra website. Accessed 28 Feb 2022, https://chopra.com.

11 CYPN website. Accessed 28 Feb 2022,
    https://www.conqueryourpcosnaturally.com.

12 Fertility Help Hub website. "Wellbeing Tips." Accessed 28 Feb 2022,
    https://www.fertilityhelphub.com/blog/wellbeing/fertility-meditation.

13 Fertility Help Hub website.

14 Fertility Help Hub website.

15 "Medication for Anxiety." Headspace. Accessed 28 Feb 2022, https://www.
    headspace.com/meditation/anxiety.

16 "Anxiety and Infertility: How to Cope." Pregnantish. Accessed 28 Feb 2022,
    https://pregnantish.com/anxiety-and-infertility-how-to-cope/.

17 "Anxiety and Infertility: How to Cope." Pregnantish.

18 "Fight or Flight Response." Psychology Tools. Accessed 28 Feb 2022,
    https://www.psychologytools.com/resource/fight-or-flight-response/.

19 "Fight or Flight Response." Psychology Tools.

20 "Medication for Anxiety." Headspace.

21 "Just 10 Minutes of Meditation Helps Anxious People Have Better Focus."
    University of Waterloo. 1 May 2017, accessed 28 Feb 2022, https://uwaterloo.
    ca/news/news/just-10-minutes-meditation-helps-anxious-people-have-better.

22 Breathworks website. What is Mindfulness. Accessed 28 Feb 2022, https://
    www.breathworks-mindfulness.org.uk/what-is-mindfulness.

23 Wikipedia. "Jon Kabat-Zinn." Accessed 28 Feb 2022, https://en.wikipedia.
    org/wiki/Jon_Kabat-Zinn.

24 Wikipedia. "Mindfulness." Accessed 28 Feb 2022, https://en.wikipedia.org/
    wiki/Mindfulness.

25 Judy Robinson. "Using Mindfulness When Dealing with Infertility." Kim
    Campbell, 20 May 2019, accessed 28 Feb 2022, https://smartfertility-
    choices.com/mindfulness-for-infertility/.

26 "Creativity is Intelligence Having Fun." Your Amazing Design blog, 21 Nov
    2017, accessed 28 Feb 2022, https://www.youramazingdesign.com/blogs/
    news/creativity-is-intelligence-having-fun-albert-einstein.

27 Gregg Braden website. Accessed 28 Feb 2022, https://www.greggbraden.com/.

28 *Science of the Heart: Exploring the Role of the Heart in Human Performance.* HeartMath Institute, online book, accessed 28 Feb 2022, https://www. heartmath.org/research/science-of-the-heart/.

29 Material from Brené Brown website, https://brenebrown.com/.

30 Material from Brené Brown website.

31 Material from Dr. Wayne W. Dyer website, https://www.drwaynedyer.com/.

32 Material from Joe Dispenza, Unlimited website.

33 Material from Kirsty Saunders website, https://www.kirstysaunders.com/.

34 Material from C. Joybell C. website, http://www.cjoybellc.com.

35 Material from Paulo Coelho's blog, https://paulocoelhoblog.com/.

36 Bronnie Ware. "The Top 5 Regrets of Dying." Accessed 28 Feb 2022, https://bronnieware.com/regrets-of-the-dying/.

37 Team Tony. "Experience the Benefits of Gratitude." Tony Robbins website, accessed 28 Feb 2022, https://www.tonyrobbins.com/health-vitality/ benefits-of-gratitude/.

38 Emmons, R.A., *Thanks!: How the New Science of Gratitude Can Make You Happier*, New York: Houghton Mifflin Company, 2007.

39 Karson McGinley. "How to Raise Your Emotional and Spiritual Vibration." Chopra, 18 Sept 2019, accessed 28 Feb 2022, https://www.chopra.com/articles/a-complete-guide-to-raise-your-vibration.

40 Emmons, R.A., *Thanks!: How the New Science of Gratitude Can Make You Happier.*

41 Author's website. https://www.sarahwilloughby.com.au/.

42 Infertility—Breaking the Silence. "Infertility and Miscarriage: Breaking the Silence, A Conversation with Laura Flynn." YouTube video, 29:53. June 12, 2020. https://www.youtube.com/watch?v=hf032y4i3wU&t=15s.

43 Olivia Fox websites, accessed 28 Feb 2022, https://www.weareoliviafox.com/, https://www.facebook.com/weareoliviafox, https://www.instagram.com/weareoliviafox/, https://www.youtube.com/channel/UC-mmb4yCpJwk7C_8fH1EhSw.

44 Thompson, Anita. "Coping with IVF, Trauma and Loss," Produced by Producer Anita Thompson. *Heartache To Hope: Coping with Infertility, IVF & Miscarriage,* Jan 17, 2022. Podcast, 39:00. https://podcasts.apple.

com/us/podcast/heartache-to-hope-coping-with-infertility-ivf-miscarriage/ id1580020269.

45 Heartache to Hope website. Accessed 28 Feb 2022, https://www.heartache2hope.net/.

46 Heartache to Hope Instagram page. Accessed 28 Feb 2022, https://www.instagram.com/heartache_2_hope/.

47 IVF Dad podcast at https://www.ivfdad.com/.

48 IVF Dad podcast.

49 Rainbow Fertility material. Accessed 28 Feb 2022, https://www.rainbowfertility.com.au/.

50 Three Little Birds Perinatal material. Accessed 28 Feb 2022, https://www.threelittlebirdsperinatal.org/.

51 SANDS material. Accessed 28 Feb 2022, https://www.sands.org.uk/.

52 SANDS material.

53 The Pink Elephant's Support Network material. Accessed 28 Feb 2022, https://www.pinkelephants.org.au/.

54 National Infertility Awareness Week material. Accessed 28 Feb 2022, https://infertilityawareness.org/.

55 Baby Loss Awareness Week material. Accessed 28 Feb 2022, https://www.babyloss-awareness.org/.

56 Harris, Colette with Carey, Dr Adam, *PCOS*, London: Thorsons, 2000.

57 Women's Health website material. Accessed 28 Feb 2022, http://www.womenshealth.gov.

58 Verity material. Accessed 28 Feb 2022, http://www.verity-pcos.org.uk.

59 Jean Hailes Women's Health material. Accessed 28 Feb 2022, http://www.jeanhailes.org.au.

60 Jean Hailes Women's Health material.

61 Jean Hailes Women's Health material.

62 PCOS symptoms are summarized from the following sources: http://www.jeanhailes.org.au, https://www.monashivf.com, https://www.betterhealth.vic.gov.au/health/conditionsandtreatments/polycystic-ovarian-syndrome-pcos, Harris, Colette with Carey, Dr Adam, *PCOS*.

63 "Polycystic Ovarian Syndrome (PCOS)," Better Health Channel, accessed 28 Feb 2022, https://www.betterhealth.vic.gov.au/health/condition-sandtreatments/polycystic-ovarian-syndrome-pcos.

A free ebook edition is available with the purchase of this book.

To claim your free ebook edition:

1. Visit MorganJamesBOGO.com
2. Sign your name CLEARLY in the space
3. Complete the form and submit a photo of the entire copyright page
4. You or your friend can download the ebook to your preferred device

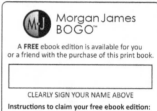

Print & Digital Together Forever.

Snap a photo

Free ebook

Read anywhere

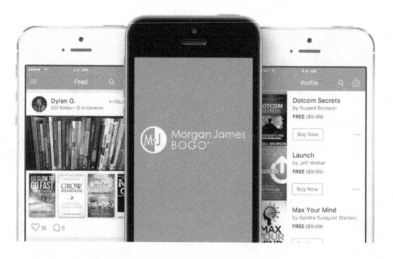

CPSIA information can be obtained
at www.ICGtesting.com
Printed in the USA
JSHW011926281022
32292JS00001B/8